Editors

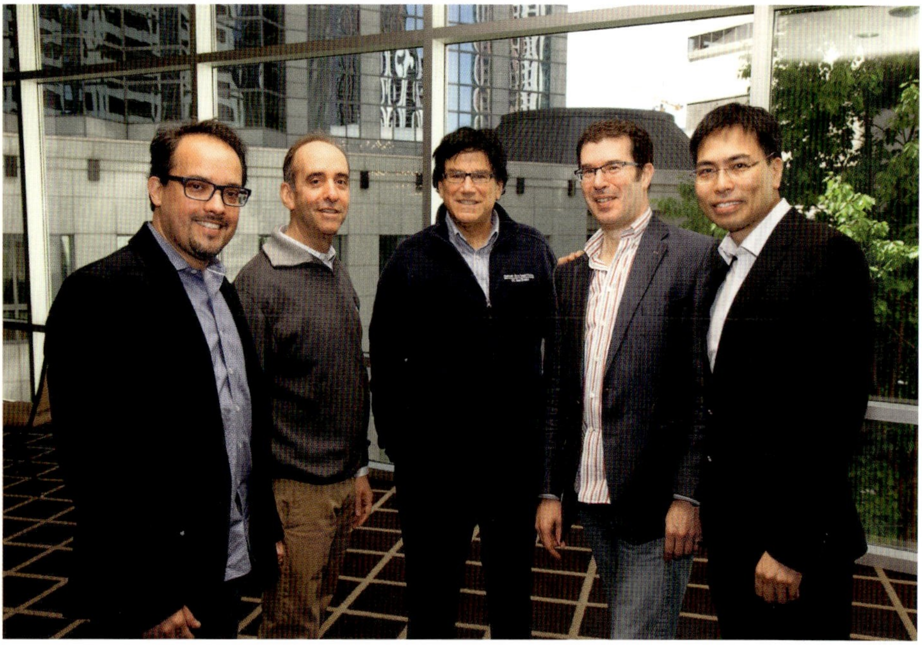

Felipe Medeiros, Jeffrey Liebmann, Robert N. Weinreb, David Garway-Heath, Christopher Leung (L-R)

DIAGNOSIS OF PRIMARY OPEN ANGLE GLAUCOMA

The 10th Consensus Report of the

World Glaucoma Association

Editors

Robert N. Weinreb
David Garway-Heath
Christopher Leung
Felipe Medeiros
Jeffrey Liebmann

Kugler Publications/Amsterdam/The Netherlands

ISBN 978-90-6299-262-1

Dirtributors:

For the USA and Canada:
American International Distribution Corporation (AIDC)
P.O. Box 2249
Williston, VT 05495
kug.orders@aidcvt.com

For all other countries:
Kugler Publications
P.O. Box 20538
1001 NM Amsterdam, The Netherlands
www.kuglerpublications.com

This publication is the tenth of a series on Consensus reports on Glaucoma under the auspices of the World Glaucoma Association

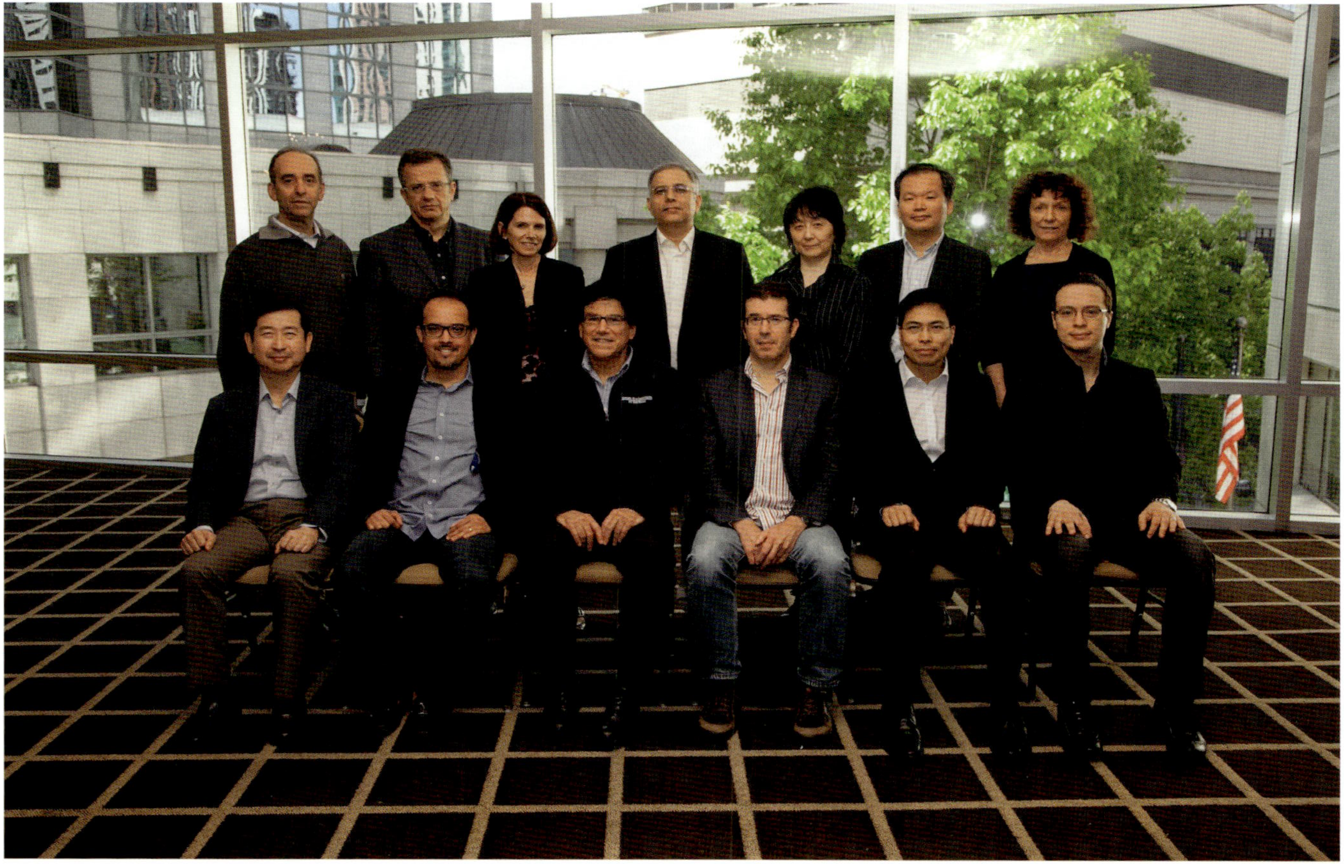

Consensus X section leaders. Top: Jeff Liebmann, Fotis Topouzis, Janey Wiggs, Tanuj Dada, Aiko Iwase, Tae-Woo Kim, Linda Zangwill
Bottom: Ki Ho Park, Felipe Medeiros, Robert N. Weinreb, David Garway-Heath, Christopher Leung, Gustavo DeMoraes

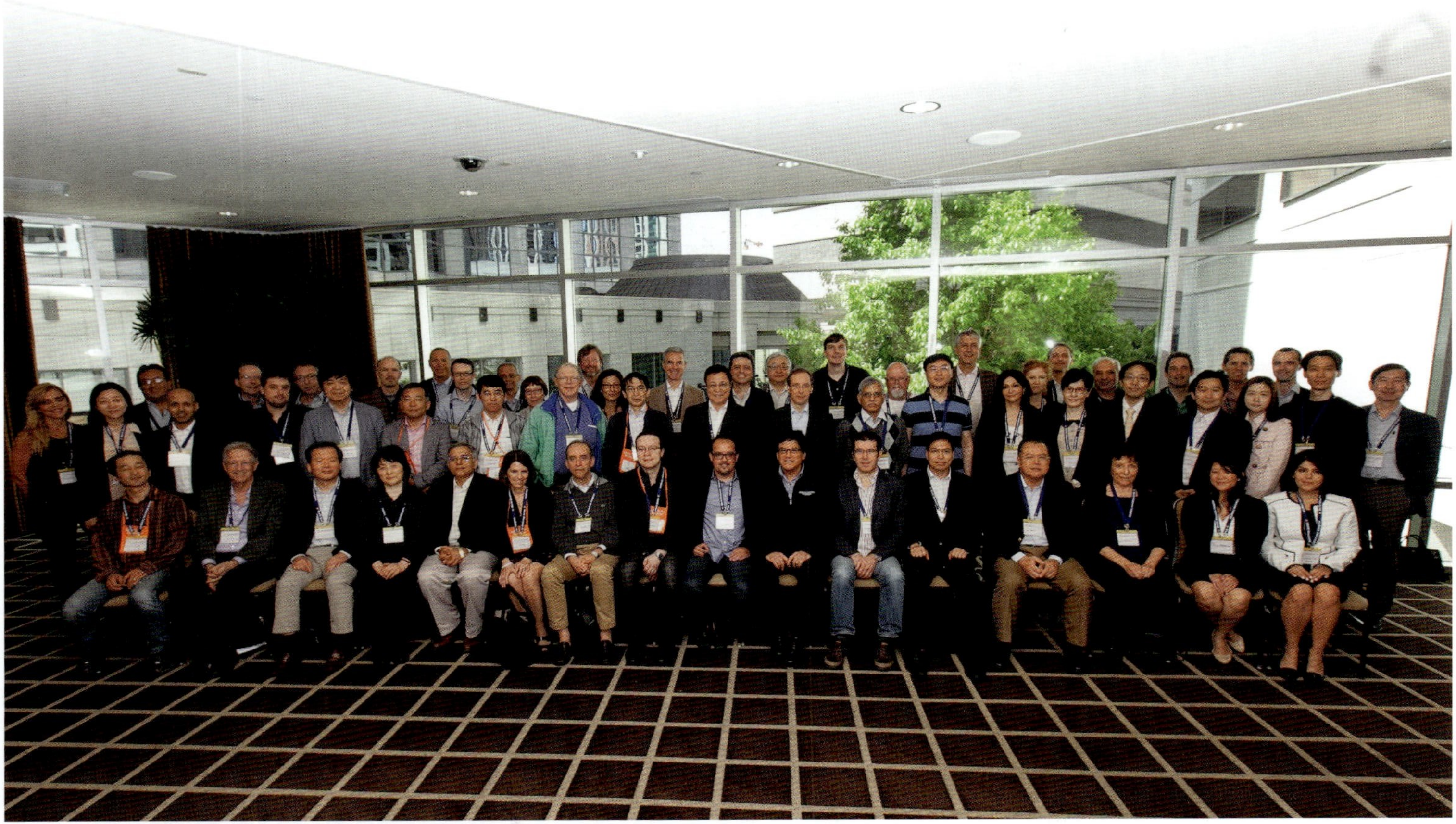

Consensus X participants

FACULTY

Consensus Initiative Chair
Robert N. Weinreb, USA

Co-chairs
David Garway-Heath, UK
Christopher Leung, Hong Kong
Felipe Medeiros, USA
Jeffrey Liebmann, USA

Section chairs
Jamie Brandt, USA
Tanuj Dada, India
Gustavo De Moraes, USA
Mingguang He, P.R. China
Aiko Iwase, Japan
Jost Jonas, Germany
Tae-Woo Kim, South Korea
Ki Ho Park, South Korea
Fotis Topouzis, Greece
Janey Wiggs, USA

Participants
Andrew, Anderson, Australia
Florent Aptel, France
Makoto Araie, Japan
Ryo Asaoka, Japan
Sanjay Asrani, USA
Tin Aung, Singapore
Augusto Azuaro-Blanco, UK
Eytan Blumenthal, Israel
Rupert Bourne, UK
Chris Bowd, USA
Alain Bron, France
Paulo Brusini, Italy
Joseph Caprioli, USA
Subho Chakrabarthi, India
Jack Cioffi, USA
Anne Louise Coleman, USA
Michael Coote, Australia
Vital Costa, Brazil
David Crabb, USA
Jonathan Crowston, Australia
Barbara Cvenkel, Slovenia
Paulus de Jong, The Netherlands
Crawford Downs, USA
Robert Fechtner, USA
Murray Fingeret, USA
John Flanagan, USA
Brad Fortune, USA
Paul Foster, UK
Panayiota Founti, Greece
Stuart Gardiner, USA
David Garway-Heath, UK
Ronnie George, India
Michael Girard, Singapore
Christopher Girkin, USA
Francisco Javier Goñi, Spain
David Greenfield, USA
Neeru Gupta, Canada
Alon Harris, USA
David Henson, UK
Donald Hood, USA
Aiko Iwase, Japan
Henry D. Jampel, USA
Chris Johnson, USA
Jost Jonas, Germany
Kenji Kashiwagi, Japan
Dan Kiage, Kenya
Tae-Woo Kim, South Korea
Miriam Kolko, Denmark

Michael, Kook, South Korea
Aravind, Krishnadas, India
Rachel Kuchtey, USA
Eun Ji Lee, South Korea
Fabian Lerner, Argentina
Christopher Leung, Hong Kong
Jeffrey Liebmann, USA
Shan Lin, USA
Vijaya Lingam, India
Catherine Liu, Taiwan
Steven Mansberger, USA
Kaweh Mansouri, Switzerland
Keith Martin, UK
Jose Martinez de la Casa, Spain
Chota Matsumoto, Japan
Allison McKendrick, Australia
Andy McNaught, Australia
Felipe Medeiros, USA
Stefano Miglior, Italy
Atsuya Miki, Japan
Sameh Mosaed, USA
Jonathan Myers, USA
Toru Nakazawa, Japan
Vinay Nangia, India
Kouros Nouri-Mahdavi, USA
Sola Olawoye, Nigeria
Augusto Paranhos, Brazil
Sung Chul Park, South Korea
Ki Ho Park, South Korea
Louis R, Pasquale, USA
Shamira Perera, Singapore
Norbert Pfeiffer, Germany
Bruce Prum, USA
Lyne Racette, USA
Pradeep Ramulu, India
Harsha Rao, India
Robert Ritch, USA
Lisandro Sakata, Brazil
Leopold, Schmetterer, Austria
Joel Schuman, USA
Chandra Sekhar, India
Ramanjit Sihoto, India
Arthur Sit, USA
George Spaeth, USA
Ingeborg Stalmans, Belgium
Kyungrim Sung, South Korea
Remo Susanna, Brasil
Akagi Tadamichi, Japan
Andrew, Tatham, UK
Christopher Teng, USA
Clement Tham, Hong Kong
Fotis Topouzis, Greece
Michael, Wall, USA
Ningli Wang, P.R. China
Ya Xing Wang, P.R. China
Roy Wilson, USA
Liang Xu, P.R. China
Xiulan Zhang, P.R. China
Linda Zangwill, USA

Recording Secretaries

Patricia Manalastas, USA
Adeleh Yarmohammadi, USA

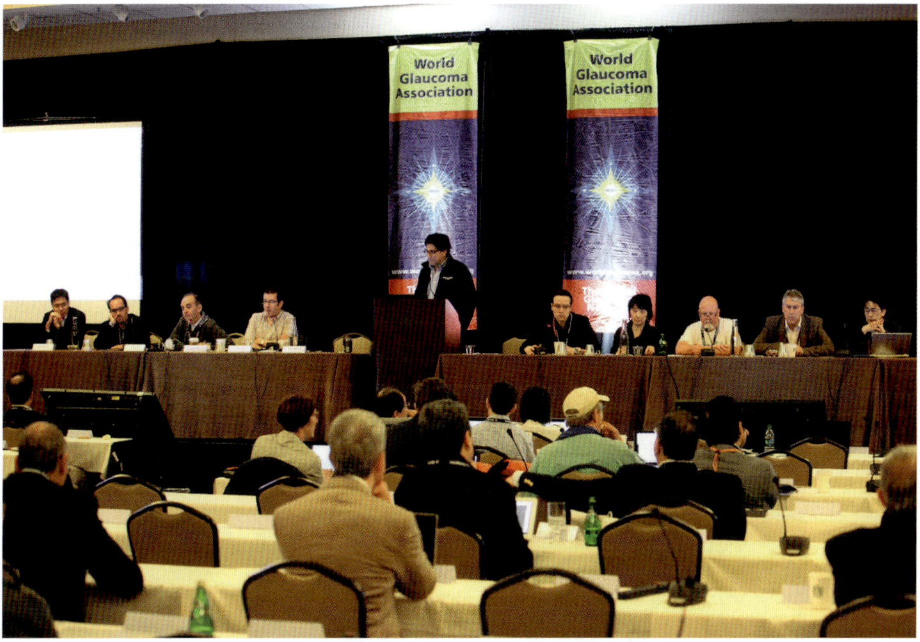

Chris Leung, Felipe Medeiros, Jeff Liebmann, David Garway-Heath and Robert N. Weinreb

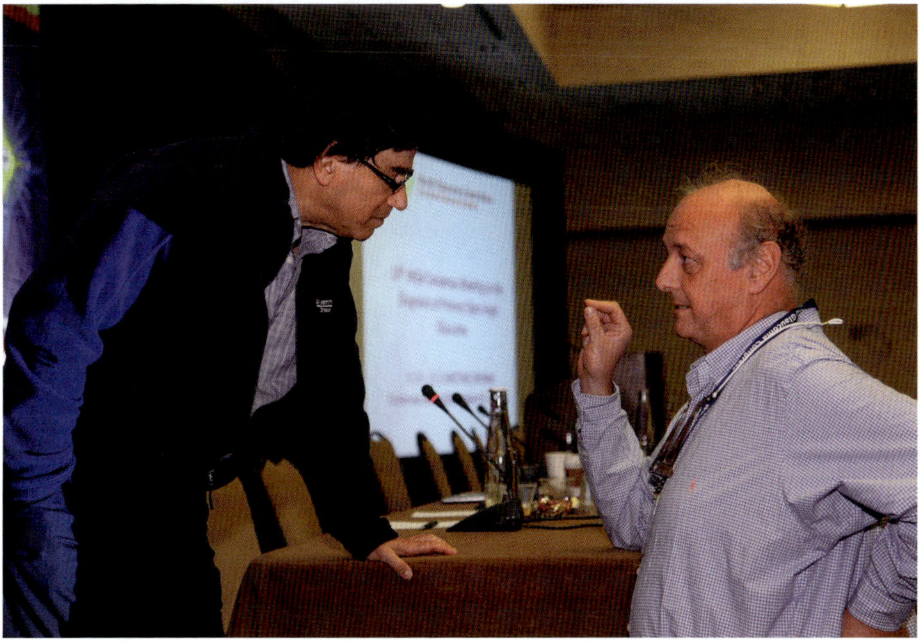

Robert N. Weinreb and Tony Hommer

WGA CONSENSUS SERIES

The Glaucoma Consensus Initiative of the World Glaucoma Association is based on the idea that the collective wisdom of a group is better than the opinion of a single expert. Assembling a sufficiently large and sufficiently diverse group of glaucoma specialists and scientists provides recommendations and insights that are likely to be superior to those of a single clinician. These recommendations and insights form the foundation for the Glaucoma Consensus Reports.

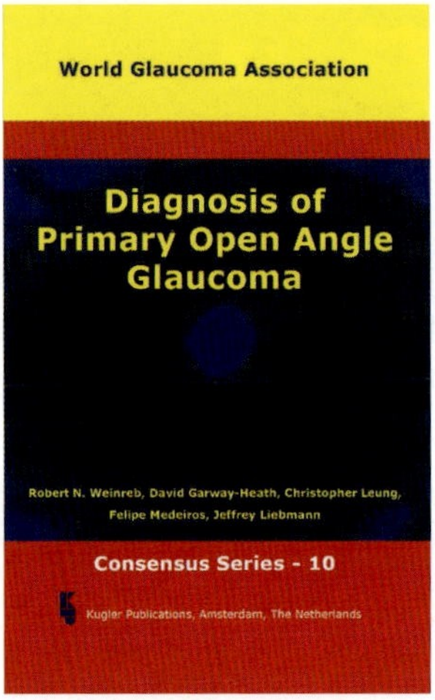

2016

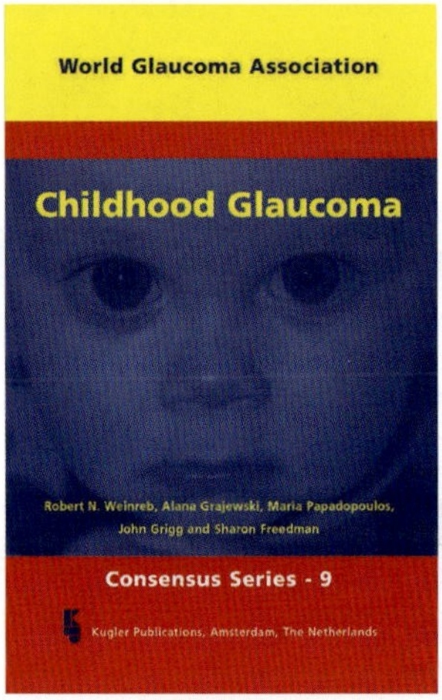

2013

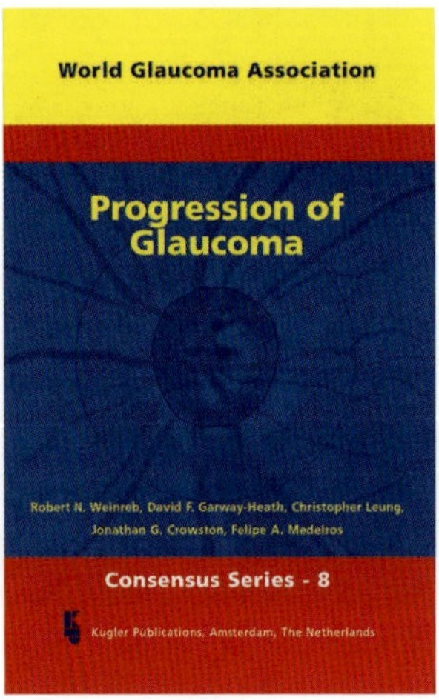

2011

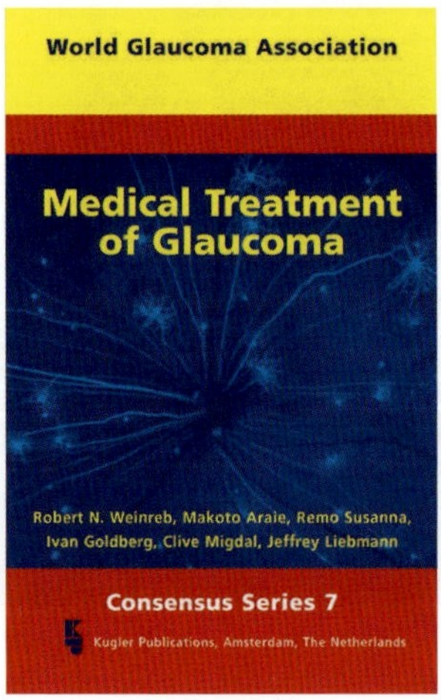

2010

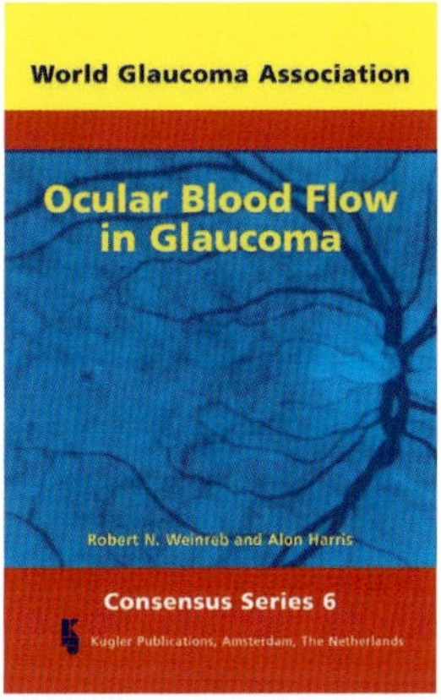

2009

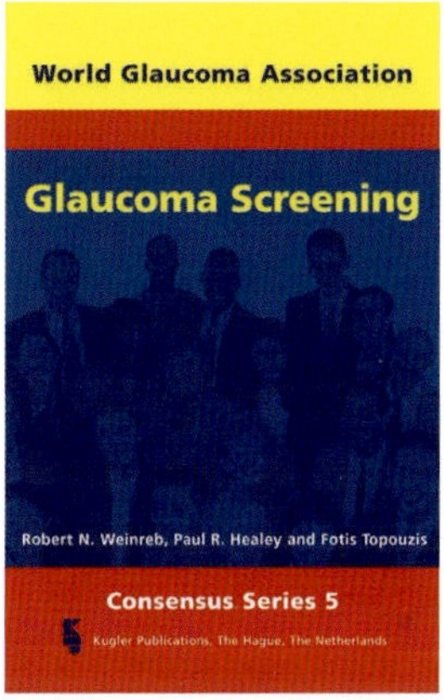

2008

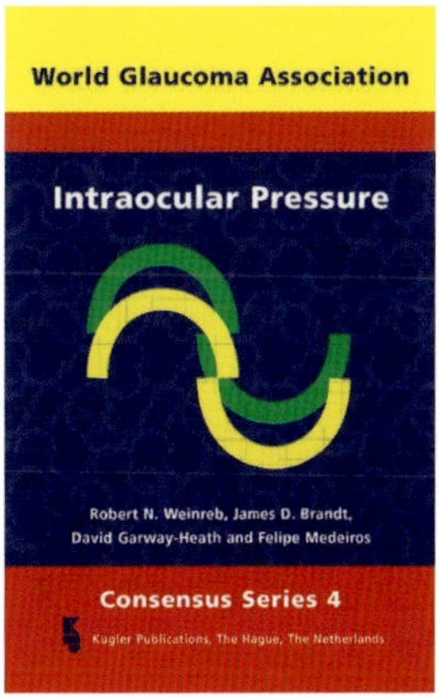

2007

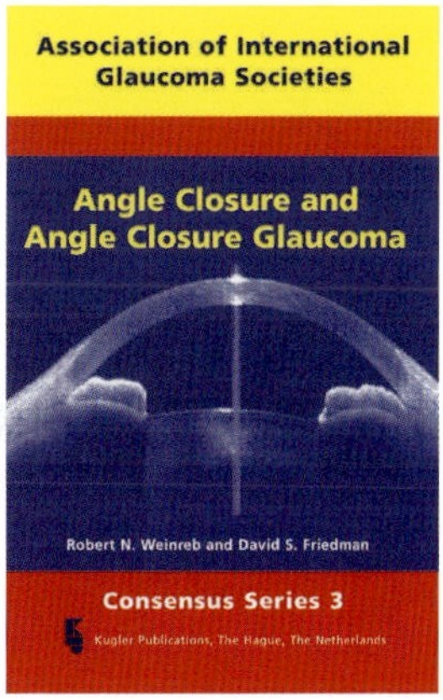

2006

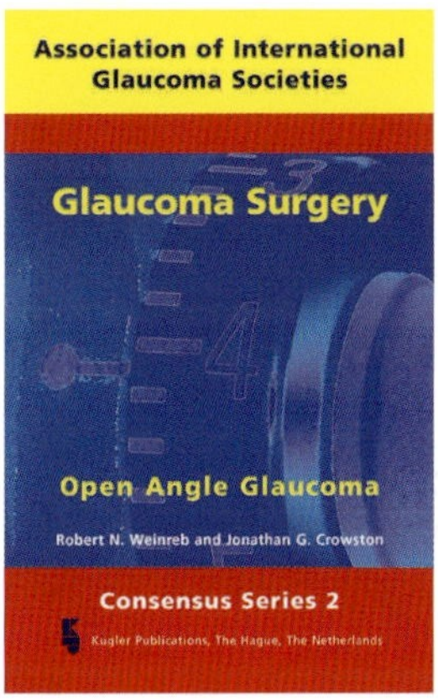

2005

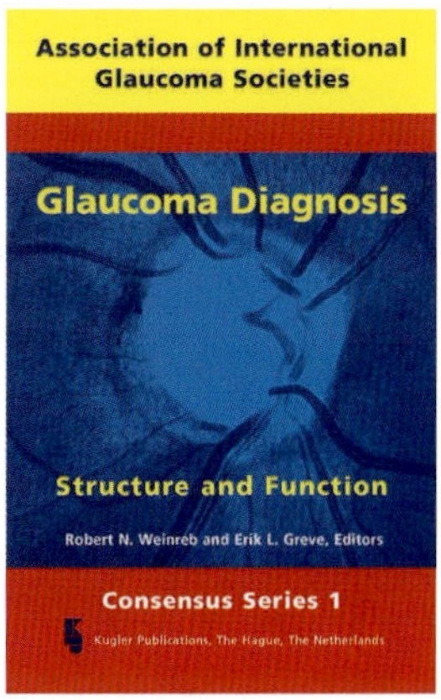

2004

CONTENTS

PREFACE

Primary Open-Angle Glaucoma was the topic of the tenth World Glaucoma Association Consensus meeting.

As with prior meetings, it was a daunting task to seek and obtain consensus on broad subject matter that ranges from diagnosis, risk profiling and screening of the disease. As it is unclear how each of us decides how we practice and the evidence to guide us often is sparse, this consensus, as well as the others, is based not only on the published literature, but also on expert opinion. Although consensus does not replace and is not a surrogate for scientific investigation, it does provide considerable value, especially when the desired evidence is lacking.

The goal of this consensus is to provide a foundation for diagnosing and managing primary open-angle glaucoma and how it can be best done in clinical practice. Identification of those areas for which we have little evidence and, therefore, the need for additional research always is a high priority. We hope that this consensus report will serve as a benchmark of our understanding. However, this consensus report is intended to be fluid. It is expected that it will be revised and improved with the emergence of new evidence.

Robert N. Weinreb, Chair

Co-chairs:

David Garway-Heath
Christopher Leung
Felipe A. Medeiros
Jeffrey Liebmann

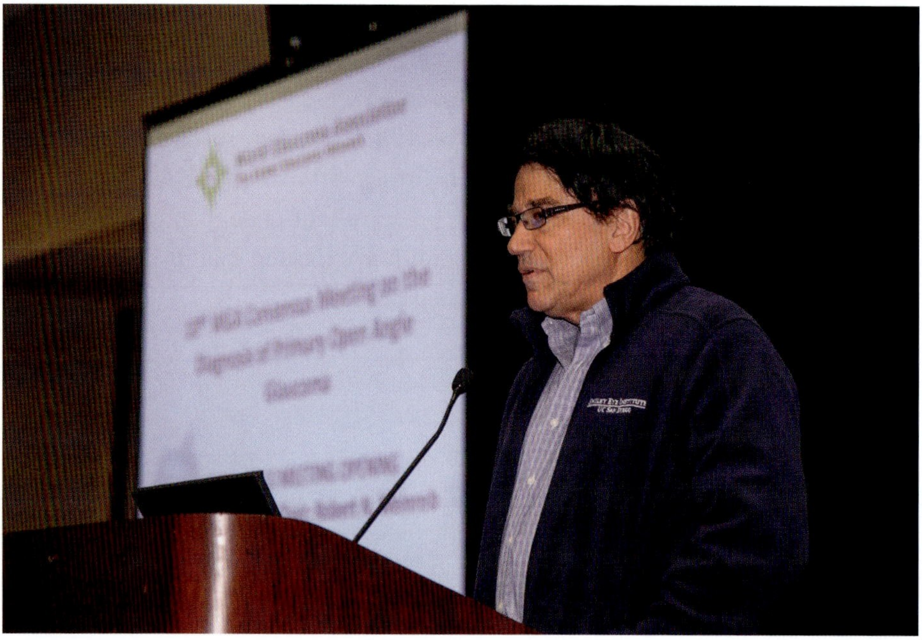

Robert N. Weinreb

INTRODUCTION

The topic for the tenth World Glaucoma Association Consensus is Primary Open-Angle Glaucoma.

Global experts were invited and assembled by our international co-Chairs, beginning in November 2015 to participate in the Forum E-Room, a unique online opportunity to facilitate discussion. Participants then were engaged in the discussion of six sections to reach consensus on key issues that permeate various aspects of primary open-angle glaucoma. The results of these thoughtful discussions then were summarized for each of the sections with preliminary consensus statements.

The Draft of the Consensus Report, including the preliminary consensus statements, was distributed to the Societies and Partners for comments prior to the Consensus Meeting that took place in Seattle on Saturday, April 30, 2016. At this time, relevant stakeholders engaged in a stimulating, educational, and thought-provoking session that reviewed and revised the consensus statements. The Consensus Report then was finalized by Consensus co-Chairs and Editors.

Robert N. Weinreb, Editor

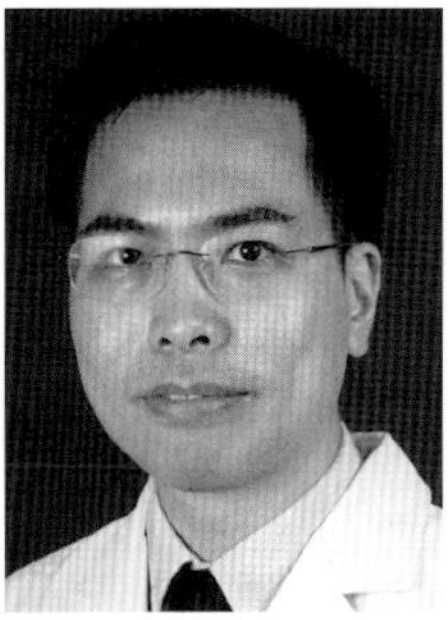

Christopher Leung

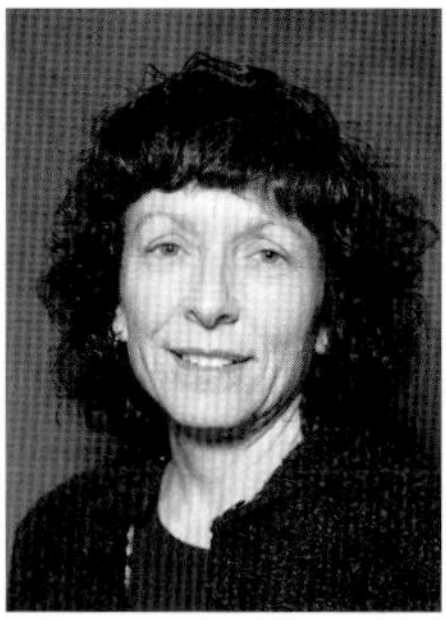

Linda Zangwill

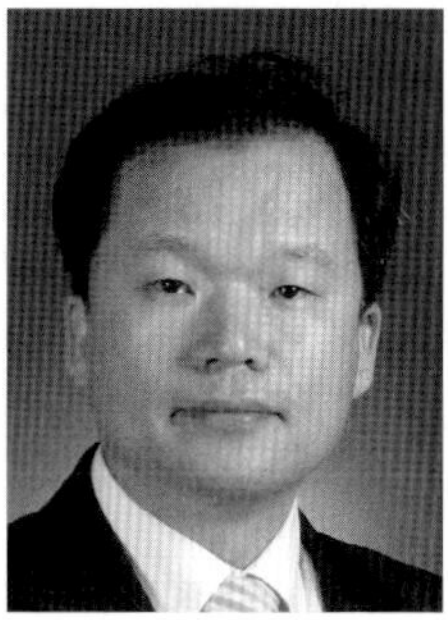

Tae-Woo Kim

1. STRUCTURE

Section leader: Christopher Leung
Section co-leaders: Linda Zangwill, Tae-Woo Kim
Contributors: Sanjay Asrani, Crawford Downs, Robert Fechtner, John Flanagan, Brad Fortune, Micheal Girard, Christopher Girkin, David Greenfield, Donald Hood, Jost Jonas, Michael Kook, Eun Ji Lee, Felipe A. Medeiros, Atsuya Miki, Toru Nakazawa, Sung Chul Park, Harsha Rao, Joel Schuman, Kyungrim Sung, Akagi Tadamichi

Consensus statements

1. Clinical evaluation and documentation of the optic nerve head is essential for the diagnosis and the monitoring of glaucoma.
2. Clinical diagnosis of glaucoma is predicated on the detection of a thinned retinal nerve fiber layer (RNFL) and narrowed neuroretinal rim.
   Comments: These features often are accompanied by deformation of the optic nerve head (ONH) (cupping).
   These features often appear first in the supero- or inferotemporal quadrants.
   Although these features are characteristic of POAG, it is important to exclude non-glaucomatous optic neuropathies.
3. Detecting progressive glaucomatous RNFL thinning and neuroretinal rim narrowing are the best currently available gold standards for glaucoma diagnosis.
   Comment: Disease-related damage should be differentiated from age-related change.
4. The diagnosis of glaucoma does not always require the detection of visual field defects with perimetry.
   Comments: Perimetric defects that correspond to structural findings increase the likelihood of glaucoma.
   Perimetry is indispensable for documentation and monitoring of functional decline in glaucoma.
5. Assessment of the color and the configuration (size and shape) of the neu-

Diagnosis of Primary Open Angle Glaucoma, pp 1-19
Edited by Robert N. Weinreb, David Garway-Heath, Christopher Leung, Felipe Medeiros, Jeffrey Liebmann

roretinal rim is important to differentiate glaucomatous from non-glaucomatous optic neuropathies.

Comment: A pale rim suggests non-glaucomatous optic neuropathy.

6. Photography is effective to document glaucomatous optic disc appearance and nerve fiber layer damage.

   Comments: Photography is particularly useful for detecting and documenting optic disc hemorrhage and rim color.

   Stereophotography is particularly useful for documenting optic disc topography.
7. Imaging technologies including optical coherence tomography (OCT), confocal scanning laser ophthalmoscopy (CSLO) and scanning laser polarimetry (SLP) provide an objective and quantitative approach to detect and monitor glaucoma.
8. OCT may be the best currently available digital imaging instrument for detecting and tracking optic nerve structural damage in glaucoma.
9. RNFL thickness is the most clinically helpful parameter of the ones currently available with OCT.

   Comments: Macular RGC loss in glaucoma also can be detected by OCT.

   RNFL thickness and macular RGC loss are complementary.

   Pitfalls of OCT such as artifacts and false segmentation should be considered when using OCT.

   GCIPL thickness (macula): The macula has the highest density of RGCs.
10. It is difficult in myopic eyes to differentiate those with and without glaucoma.

    Comments: In myopic eyes, documented progressive optic neuropathy can be used to make the differential diagnosis of glaucoma.

    Reference databases do not currently include highly myopic eyes and, therefore, are not appropriate for diagnosing RNFL damage in them.

1.1. Clinical diagnosis of glaucoma

1.1.1. Assessment of the retinal nerve fiber layer and neuroretinal rim

Glaucomatous optic neuropathy is an axonopathy, where damage to the visual pathway is driven by insult to retinal ganglion cell (RGC) axons as they exit the eye at the optic nerve head (ONH).[1,2] The lamina cribrosa has been considered to be the principal site of RGC axonal damage in human glaucoma.[3-5] Clinical detection of RGC axonal damage largely consists in red-free retinal nerve fiber layer (RNFL) photography and optical coherence tomography (OCT) imaging of the RNFL.[6-10] While all forms of optic neuropathies exhibit RGC loss and RNFL thinning, glaucoma is unique in demonstrating also progressive narrowing of the neuroretinal rim.[11-14] RNFL defects and neuroretinal rim loss are typically located at the inferotemporal and superotemporal sectors of the ONH. As the RNFL and the neuroretinal rim are largely composed of the axons of RGCs, detecting progressive RNFL thinning and neuroretinal rim narrowing has been suggested to the best available reference standard for glaucoma diagnosis in the 2004 World Glaucoma Association Consensus meeting.[15] However, recent evidence suggests that progressive RNFL thinning and neuroretinal rim narrowing can also be detected in normal healthy individuals.[16,17] It has been estimated that the mean rate of change of average RNFL thickness measured by a spectral-domain OCT in normal healthy eyes was -0.52 μm/year [95% confidence interval (CI), -0.86 to -0.17], after controlling for covariates.[16] Younger individuals were associated with a faster rate of RNFL thinning. In another study examining progressive neuroretinal rim narrowing measured by a CSLO, the rate of change of global neuroretinal rim area was -2.1 mm^2/year (95% CI, -4.2 to -0.02) for healthy subjects of African descent and -2.3 mm^2/year (95% CI, -4.9 to 0.3) for healthy subjects of European descent.[17] In other words, detecting progressive RNFL thinning and progressive neuroretinal rim narrowing may not necessarily imply the development or progression of glaucoma. In a prospective study following 150 eyes of 90 glaucoma patients at four-month intervals for a mean of 3.8 years, 50.0%, 30.0% and 27.3% of eyes showed progression by trend analyses of the inner macular, total macular and circumpapillary RNFL thicknesses, respectively.[18] After accounting for age-related changes, the proportions of eyes detected with progression decreased to 20.0%, 16.0% and 26.7%, respectively. Differentiating age-related from disease-related RNFL/ONH changes is relevant to the diagnosis and monitoring of glaucoma.

1.1.2. Assessment of the lamina cribrosa and the ONH surface

Although objective evaluation of ONH deformation or cupping can be challenging with slit-lamp or photographic examination of the optic disc, Fourier-domain OCT (FD-OCT) has facilitated measurements of the deformation of the lamina cribrosa and the ONH surface.[19] Laminar depth is significantly larger in glaucoma patients with younger age, higher untreated IOP, and lower RNFL thickness as measured with OCT.[20] Several studies have linked changes in the appearance of the lamina cribrosa (focal defects) in OCT images to glaucomatous damage,[21-25] and at least one study has linked longitudinal change in the peripheral lamina cribrosa to optic disc hemorrhage.[26] Further, persistent reversal of laminar cupping after trabeculectomy is correlated with reduced rates of glaucoma progression.[27] In a long-term, prospective study, progressive posterior deformation of the anterior lamina cribrosa surface and the ONH surface was found in glaucoma patients and the degree of deformation was associated with the mean intraocular pressure during study follow-up.[28] These studies underscore the importance of evaluating the deformation and alteration of ONH and lamina cribrosa for glaucoma evaluation although measurement of ONH and lamina cribrosa deformation per se is unlikely to be sufficient to establish a diagnosis of glaucomatous optic neuropathy.

1.2. Role of perimetry in glaucoma diagnosis

Histological studies have shown that RGC loss is evident in human glaucoma before visual field sensitivity declines in automated testing.[29,30] Structural changes of the ONH and the RNFL detected in clinical examination and/or digital imaging of the ONH/RNFL often precede detectable changes in the visual field measured by standard automated white-on-white perimetry and a number of studies have reported progressive ONH/RNFL changes to be predictive of subsequent development of visual field loss. Medeiros and colleagues followed 407 glaucoma suspects – eyes with a history of IOP > 21 mmHg and/or a glaucomatous appearance of the optic disc but without visual field defects at the baseline examination – for a mean of 8.0 years and showed that progressive optic disc changes detected by stereophotographs was 25.8 times (95% confidence interval: 16.0-14.7) more likely to develop visual field defects during follow-up.[31] Using the CSLO to measure the neuroretinal rim area for 328 patients with suspected glaucoma with each patient having a minimum of five CSLO examinations during a minimum of two years of follow-up, the authors reported in another study that each 0.01 mm^2/year faster rate of rim area loss was associated with a 2.94 times higher risk of development of visual field defects.[14] Chuahan and colleagues imaged the ONH with the CSLO and standard automated perimetry every six months for 81 open-angle glaucoma patients over a median of 11.0 years and demonstrated that ONH surface depression, analyzed with Topographic Change Analysis, is predictive of subsequent visual field progression.[32] In a prospective study following 139 primary-open angle glaucoma patients at ~four-month intervals over five years, Yu and colleagues showed that progressive RNFL thinning determined by event-based (Guided Progression Analysis – GPA) and trend-based (Trend-based Progression Analysis – TPA) analysis of the RNFL thickness maps captured by the spectral-domain OCT was associated with > five-fold and > eight-fold increases in risk of subsequent development of visual field progression, respectively.[33] Notably, in the Ocular Hypertension Treatment Study (OHTS) in which primary open-angle glaucoma end-point was determined by changes in the VF or optic disc, 40 eyes reached only a visual field end-point (87 eyes reached an optic disc end point).[34] Although the OHTS suggests either visual field or optic disc may show the first evidence of glaucomatous damage, it is worth noting the optic disc end-point was determined by subjective evaluation of optic disc photographs taken once a year. As visual field defects can also develop in non-glaucomatous optic neuropathy and macular diseases, examination of the optic disc and the RNFL is always necessary to establish a diagnosis of glaucoma.

1.3. How to differentiate glaucomatous from non-glaucomatous optic neuropathies?

The clinical distinction between glaucomatous from non-glaucomatous optic neuropathies can be subtle and is largely based upon the assessment of the color and morphology of the neuroretinal rim.[35-37] A pale neuroretinal rim suggests optic neuropathy other than glaucoma, whereas progressive neuroretinal rim narrowing and ONH deformation signifies glaucomatous damage. Neuroretinal rim pallor was found to be 94% specific for non-glaucomatous optic neuropathy, whereas focal or diffuse obliteration of the neuroretinal rim was 87% specific for glaucomatous optic neuropathy.[36] Rim pallor in excess of cupping was reported to be 90% specific for non-glaucomatous optic neuropathy in a study including glaucoma patients with normal intraocular pressure and patients with intracranial mass lesions.[37] Glaucomatous optic discs may appear pale in the late stages because the loss of neuroretinal rim is extensive. The lamina cribrosa is exposed in advanced glaucoma (light reflected from the lamina cribrosa is whitish), rendering the optic discs (not neuroretinal rim) pale-looking.

1.4. Imaging technologies for detection of glaucoma

Although optic disc photographs remains important in the evaluation of the ONH, imaging technologies including OCT, confocal scanning laser ophthalmoscopy (CSLO) and scanning laser polarimetry (SLP) have provided a quantitative and objective approach to detect and monitor glaucoma. FD-OCT has gained popularity over CSLO and SLP because of its higher scan speed, higher image resolution, and being able to quantify both the RNFL and ONH parameters. Measurement of the ganglion cell layer and inner plexiform layer thickness is also feasible with OCT. Although OCT has been reported to have high diagnostic performance for glaucoma detection,[38-41] there are limitations in OCT measurements. RNFL thickness measurements are influenced by the signal-to-noise ratio of the OCT images.[42,43] In addition, artifacts including epiretinal membrane,[44] retinoschisis,[45,46] vitreous opacity,[47] and false segmentation can lead to errorous measurements.[48] The circumpapillary RNFL thickness is also affected by the scan circle location[49,50] and head tilt.[51] Such pitfalls should be considered when interpretating OCT measurements.

1.4.1. RNFL thickness

RNFL thickness maps provide visualization and quantitative measurement RNFL thickness information throughout the peripapillary retina from OCT ONH volume/cube scans. RNFL thickness deviation maps use reference databases to provide spatial information on the pattern and probability of ONH RNFL damage. In contrast to RNFL thickness profile measurements along a circumpapillary circle (cpRNFL), RNFL deviation maps provide spatial information on the defect size, shape, and location of RNFL damage. Relying on cpRNFL can miss RNFL damage that is outside the circumpapillary measurement; RNFL maps overcome this limitation, and have the advantage of facilitating visualization of the focal wedge shaped defects.

Several studies show that RNFL thickness deviation maps have higher diagnostic sensitivity for glaucoma detection at a high level of specificity compared with circumpapillary RNFL measurements.[52-55] Specifically, standardized scoring of RNFL thickness deviation maps based on the defect size, shape, depth, location, and distance from the optic disc had similar sensitivity (95.0%) to circumpapillary RNFL thickness criteria of one clock-hour outside normal limits at the 5% level (93.4%), but specificity of the RNFL map was significantly higher (95.1% vs. 83.3%, $P < 0.001$).[51,55] One study showed that RNFL deviation maps area under receiver operating characteristic curve (AUC) performed significantly better at detecting localized RNFL defects compared with clock-hour circumpapillary RNFL thickness (AUC: 0.94 vs. 0.86, respectively[53]), while another did not show a difference between RNFL map evaluated using a qualitative semi-quantitative continuous cluster metric and cpRNFL thickness pattern deviation (AUC: 0.74 vs 0.72, respectively).[55]

1.4.2. Neuroretinal rim width

Recent improvements in OCT retinal layer segmentation has facilitated the development of a new neuroretinal rim summary measure, minimimum rim width (MRW), defined as the miminum distance between Bruch's membrane opening (BMO) and the internal limiting membrane (ILM).[56] The MRW has been shown to have better diagnostic accuracy for differentiating between glaucoma and healthy eyes that standard neuroretinal rim measurements.[57-61]

Evidence suggests that the diagnostic accuracy for glaucoma detection of MRW is better than neuroretinal area, and similar or better than RNFL thickness.[57,62,63] However, results vary by severity of disease and there is some evidence that RNFL thickness may be more sensitive for detection of early glaucomatous damage.[60]

It is important to note that in eyes with gamma zone parapapillary atrophy (PPA in areas of the optic disc without intact Bruch's membrane), Bruch's membrane does not extend to the margin of the optic nerve scleral canal, and that in these eyes, the distance between the end of Bruch's membrane and the nearest surface represents more the thickness of the RNFL than the width of the rim. Many myopic eyes have gamma zone PPA.[64] For this reason, in eyes with parapapillary gamma zone the MRW should be interpreted with caution.

The angle from the fovea and the center of the optic disc measured as the BMO center has been shown to affect the MRW and the pattern of RNFL thickness.[57,65-67] Correcting for the disc to foveal angle reduces the variability of measures across eyes and can improve the diagnostic accuracy of these measurements.[57,66,67]

1.4.3. Ganglion cell and inner plexiform layer thickness at the macula

The macula has the highest density of RGCs. Glaucomatous damage to the macula is relatively common, and can be measured as loss of the ganglion cell layer, macular RNFL, and inner plexiform layers.[68] Loss of these three layers, in combination or individually can be measured using OCT. It is most common to measure the ganglion cell layer (GCL) and inner plexiform layer (IPL) together as it is often challenging to accurately segment the GCL and IPL separately, and recent evidence suggests that the diagnostic accuracy of the GCL separately is similar to that of the combination of the GCL and IPL (GCIPL). Macular damage/RGC loss can occur relatively early in glaucoma, and can be missed and/or underestimated when standard visual tests such as the 24-2 test are utilized.[68-70] It should be noted that macular scans of the ganglion cell complex are difficult to interpret in eyes with macula pathology including macular edema, age-related macular degeneration and other age-related eye diseases that are common co-morbidities in eyes with glaucoma.

The preponderance of evidence published to date indicates that OCT scans of the macula have equal or lower diagnostic power for glaucoma detection as compared to peripapillary (circumpapillary) RNFL thickness profiles. Specifically, a recent Cochrane review compared the diagnostic accuracy of macular parameters, specifically the ganglion cell complex (GCC) and ganglion cell IPL (GCIPL), with the accuracy of RNFL parameters for detecting manifest glaucoma.[71] Based on a review of 36 studies, the authors conclude that "RNFL parameters are still preferable to macular parameters for diagnosing manifest glaucoma, but the differences are small." The conclusions are not generalizable to glaucoma patients with high myopia, tilted discs or other possible co-moribidities. This is true regardless of which macular retinal layers are measured (the GCL, the macular RNFL, the GCIPL, etc.). Moreover, obtaining reliable measurements of RNFL thickness requires review of only two image feature boundaries/segmentations, whereas meaningful macular retinal layer thickness measurements and thus many more image segmentations to review, an increased burden on patients, clinic staff and physicians.

It is important to note that studies comparing macula and RNFL thickness measurements have been based on cpRNFL profiles and not RNFL thickness maps; cpRNFL profiles that can miss RNFL damage in some eyes that are detectable on RNFL thickness maps. Moreover, the general metrics used for analyzing circumpapillary (cp)RNFL thickness and macular thickness (GCC, GCPIL/RGC+ etc.) are not necessarily the most sensitive metric to detect damage. While past studies have shown little difference in sensitivity/specificity between cpRNFL and macular measures, there is evidence in some eyes, macular scans will detect macular damage missed by cpRNFL analysis, while in other eyes macular scans will miss damage outside the region of the macular scan.[69,72] Better metrics that focus on regions of interest show promise for improving the diagnostic value of these measures.[73] In addition, there is evidence that combining data from RNFL and macula scan can improve glaucoma detection.[74]

A limitation of all structural measures is that they reach a floor effect at which point residual thickness from non-neural tissue contributes to the measurement and thinning due to glaucoma can no longer be detected. For example, at the measurement floor, RNFL, thickness from blood vessels and glial cells and not necessarily neural tissue are contributing to the measurement of RNFL thickness, and it is no longer diagnostic. GCIPL measurements have a similar problem, but the floor is reached later in the disease. It should also be noted that there is significant age-related loss in healthy subjects,[66,75] so that adjusting for age is important in the interpretation of structural measures for glaucoma detection.

1.4.4. Lamina cribrosa and ONH surface depth

The lamina cribrosa is a sieve-like structure that provides support to RGC axons and retinal blood vessels as they exit the eye through the scleral canal to the retrobulbar cerebrospinal space.[4] Although the pathophysiology of glaucoma is not fully understood, there is evidence that remodeling of the lamina cribrosa is associated with glaucomatous axonal loss such as a RNFL defect, and neuroretinal rim thinning/notching.[25,76]

Moreover, reports have demonstrated significant correlation between morphologic features of the lamina cribrosa such as depth, thickness, or focal defects and the severity or progression of glaucoma.[3,24,77-86] Until recently, attenuation of the OCT signal as it penetrates into deep layers has prevented *in-vivo* visualization of deep tissues such as the lamina cribrosa. Recent advances in swept-source (SS) OCT and enhanced depth imaging (EDI) SD-OCT has provided increased penetration of the OCT signal with visualization and quantification of the lamina cribrosa achievable *in-vivo* in many patients.[83,85-91]

Focal lamina cribrosa defects, often defined as a laminar hole or laminar disinsertions violating the normal U- or W-shaped contour of the anterior laminar surface,[22,24,26,92] can be reproducibly detected by qualitative review of SS-OCT and EDI SD-OCT images. Although detection of focal damage is subjective and time consuming, good inter-observer reproducibility is achievable using standardized protocols.[76,92] The anterior border of the lamina cribrosa is visible in most eyes, while the posterior border of the lamina cribrosa is rarely detectable with current imaging modalities.[83]

The anterior lamina cribrosa surface depth has been suggested as a robust quantitative measure of lamina cribrosa remodeling and displacement.[93] Anterior lamina cribrosa surface depth is measured from the BMO to the anterior surface of lamina cribrosa using manual and semi-automated[94,96] and fully automated methods.[97] Anterior lamina cribrosa surface depth varies with severity of disease.[98] In addition, the magnitude of laminar remodeling measured as anterior lamina cribrosa surface depth is greater in younger eyes compared to older eyes, and varies by race suggesting that its relationship with glaucomatous structural and functional may show considerable variability across eyes.[96] Moreover, there is consistent evidence that the anterior lamina cribrosa surface depth changes with IOP. Specifically Lee *et al.*[93] showed that the posterior displacement of the lamina cribrosa measured was significantly decreased after IOP was lowered after both medical and surgical interventions. In addition, Belghith *et al.*[97] demonstrated changes in anterior lamina cribrosa surface depth are strongly associated with changes in IOP over time.

ONH surface depth changes measured using CSLO have been shown to occur before RNFL thinning.[28,98] ONH surface depth can also be measured using OCT and has been shown, along with lamina cribrosa surface depth to be displaced anteriorly as well as posteriorly relative to the BMO and is related to age and IOP.[28]

Although there is evidence that the anterior cribrosa surface depth and ONH surface depth are associated with glaucoma damage, there is insufficient evidence that these measurements are clinically useful; large-scale studies are necessary. Additional limitations to using anterior lamina cribrosa surface depth for glaucoma management include: (1) limited visibility of anterior lamina cribrosa surface due to insufficient signal penetration, shadowing of retinal blood vessels and neuroretinal rim tissue obscuring visualization in some patients; (2) strong association with IOP, race and age; and (3) lack of instrument software for automated measurement. Limitations of using ONH surface depth for clinical management of glaucoma include lack of instrument software for automated measurement and its association with IOP and age.

1.5. Glaucoma diagnosis in eyes with myopia

Detecting RNFL defects, neuroretinal rim loss, and ONH deformation in eyes with myopia is often challenging in clinical examination. The higher prevalence of tilted disc and peripapillary atrophy in myopic eyes also renders digitial imaging technologies less effective to measure the neuroretinal rim configuration and the RNFL thickness. It has been consistently shown that the specificity for detection of RNFL abnormalities is low in both time-domain and FD-OCT.[99-105] This is in part attributed to the fact that myopic eyes exhibit a different spatial distribution of the RNFL bundles and that the normative databases of most OCT instruments do not have reference measurements obtained from eyes with moderate or high myopia. The inferotemporal and superotemporal RNFL fiber bundles in myopic eyes often converge towards the macula, rendering the RNFL at the superior and inferior quadrants relatively thin compared with non-myopic eyes.[106] A recent study indicates that the inclusion of a myopic normative database can significantly improve the specificity of OCT for detection of RNFL abnormalities in eyes with high myopia without compromising the sensitivity.[107] Alternatively, documenting progressive changes of the RNFL and the neuroretinal rim is also useful to make the differential diagnosis of glaucoma.

1.6. ONH biomechanics

While IOP is a major risk factor for glaucoma and IOP-lowering is the only proven treatment for the disease, the mechanism of glaucomatous optic nerve injury is not well understood. ONH biomechanics, which are the physical manifestations of the IOP force distribution in the tissues, are thought to be important to glaucoma pathophysiology.[3-5] However, no studies to date have directly linked ONH biomechanics to disease in human patients, or elucidated the pathways through which IOP-induced mechanical strain damages the RGC axons as they pass through the ONH. The ONH is of particular interest from a biomechanical perspective because it is a weak spot within an otherwise strong corneo-scleral envelope. The lamina cribrosa provides structural and functional support to the RGC axons as they pass from the relatively high-pressure environment in the eye to a low-pressure region in the retrobulbar cerebrospinal space.[1,2] To protect the RGCs in this unique anatomic region, the lamina cribrosa in higher primates has developed into a complex structure composed of a three-dimensional (3D) network of flexible, load-bearing beams of connective tissue that encase the capillaries feeding the laminar region. The peripapillary sclera provides the mechanical boundary conditions for the ONH, in that forces and deformation are transmitted to the lamina cribrosa through its insertion in the scleral canal wall. Hence, the structural stiffness of the peripapillary sclera influences how the lamina deforms, and the lamina and sclera act as a structural system to withstand IOP.[5,108,109] Axoplasmic transport blockade in the ONH has been associated with acute[110,111] and chronic IOP elevations,[112] which indicates that IOP and its mechanical effects on the load-bearing tissues, vasculature,[113,114] and/or cells directly affects axonal homeostasis.

Early glaucomatous damage has not been rigorously studied in humans because human cadaver eyes with well-characterized early damage are rare and definitive glaucoma diagnosis in patients generally occurs after considerable damage has occurred. There are several findings in the nonhuman primate (NHP) model of glaucoma that yield evidence that biomechanical biomarkers may exist, however. Following moderate experimental IOP elevations in NHPs, the following changes in ONH and peripapillary scleral connective tissue architecture and material properties have been described at the onset of confocal scanning laser tomography-detected ONH surface change (clinical cupping): (1) enlargement and elongation of the neural canal;[115] (2) posterior deformation and thickening of the lamina cribrosa;[116] (3) outward migration of the posterior lamina insertion point and significant but less pronounced outward migration of the anterior lamina insertion point;[117] (4) alterations in the elastic and viscoelastic material properties of the peripapillary sclera.[118,119] These data strongly support the notion that connective tissue remodeling and new connective tissue synthesis are very active in this early stage of the neuropathy, which may serve as future imaging-based biomechanical biomarkers of disease. Furthermore, the lamina cribrosa migrates posteriorly in the neural canal during glaucomatous progression in NHPs, and that process starts early in the disease.[117]

Ideally, glaucoma diagnostic techniques would identify the majority of patients that require treatment early in the disease course and rule out glaucoma in suspects that would not otherwise progress to vision loss. While these studies lend credence to the notion that ONH biomechanics underlie a significant portion of glaucoma etiology, the available data do not definitively link ONH biomechanical behavior to glaucoma pathogenesis and progression. Hence, diagnosis of glaucoma based on a biomechanical biomarker(s) has yet to be developed and proven in patients.

References

1. Zeimer RC, Ogura Y. The relation between glaucomatous damage and optic nerve head mechanical compliance. Arch Ophthalmol 1989;107:1232-1234.
2. Downs JC, Roberts MD, Burgoyne CF. Mechanical environment of the optic nerve head in glaucoma. Optom Vis Sci 2008;85:425-435.
3. Quigley HA, Addicks EM. Regional differences in the structure of the lamina cribrosa and their relation to glaucomatous optic nerve damage. Arch Ophthalmol 1981;99:137-143.
4. Zeimer R. Biomechanical Properties of the Optic Nerve Head. In: Drance SM (Ed), Optic Nerve in Glaucoma, pp. 107-121. Amsterdam/New York: Kugler Publications 1995.
5. Downs JC. Optic nerve head biomechanics in aging and disease. Exp Eye Res 2015;133:19-29.
6. Quigley HA, Miller NR, George T. Clinical evaluation of nerve fiber layer atrophy as an indi-

cator of glaucomatous optic nerve damage. Arch Ophthalmol 1980;98:1564-1571.
7. Quigley HA, Addicks EM. Quantitative studies of retinal nerve fiber layer defects. Arch Ophthalmol 1982;100:807-814.
8. Suh MH, Kim DM, Kim YK, Kim TW, Park KH. Patterns of progression of localized retinal nerve fibre layer defect on red-free fundus photographs in normal-tension glaucoma. Eye (Lond) 2010;24:857-863.
9. Leung CK, Yu M, Weinreb RN, et al. Retinal nerve fiber layer imaging with spectral-domain optical coherence tomography: patterns of retinal nerve fiber layer progression. Ophthalmology 2012;119:1858-1866.
10. Xu G, Weinreb RN, Leung CK. Retinal nerve fiber layer progression in glaucoma: a comparison between retinal nerve fiber layer thickness and retardance. Ophthalmology 2013;120:2493-500.
11. Airaksinen PJ, Drance SM. Neuroretinal rim area and retinal nerve fiber layer in glaucoma. Arch Ophthalmol 1985;103:203-204.
12. Airaksinen PJ, Drance SM, Douglas GR, Schulzer M. Neuroretinal rim areas and visual field indices in glaucoma. Am J Ophthalmol 1985;99:107-110.
13. Jonas JB, Fernández MC, Stürmer J. Pattern of glaucomatous neuroretinal rim loss. Ophthalmology 1993;100:63-68.
14. Medeiros FA, Lisboa R, Zangwill LM, et al. Evaluation of progressive neuroretinal rim loss as a surrogate end point for development of visual field loss in glaucoma. Ophthalmology 2014;121:100-109.
15. Coleman A, Friedman D, Gandolfi S, Singh K, Tuulonen A. Levels of evidence of diagnostic studies. In: Weinreb RN, Greve EL (Eds.), Glaucoma diagnosis: Structure and function, pp. 9-12. Consensus series I. Amsterdam: Kugler Publications 2004.
16. Leung CK, Yu M, Weinreb RN, et al. Retinal nerve fiber layer imaging with spectral-domain optical coherence tomography: a prospective analysis of age-related loss. Ophthalmology 2012;119:731-737.
17. Hammel N, Belghith A, Bowd C, et al. Rate and Pattern of Rim Area Loss in Healthy and Progressing Glaucoma Eyes. Ophthalmology 2016;123:760-770.
18. Leung CK, Ye C, Weinreb RN, et al. Impact of age-related change of retinal nerve fiber layer and macular thicknesses on evaluation of glaucoma progression. Ophthalmology 2013;120:2485-2492.
19. Kim TW, Kagemann L, Girard MJ, et al. Imaging of the lamina cribrosa in glaucoma: perspectives of pathogenesis and clinical applications. Curr Eye Res 2013;38:903-909.
20. Jung KI, Jung Y, Park KT, Park CK. Factors affecting plastic lamina cribrosa displacement in glaucoma patients. Invest Ophthalmol Vis Sci 2014;55:7709-7715.
21. Abe RY, Gracitelli CP, Diniz-Filho A, Tatham AJ, Medeiros FA. Lamina Cribrosa in Glaucoma: Diagnosis and Monitoring. Current Ophthalmology Reports 2015;3:74-84.
22. Faridi OS, Park SC, Kabadi R, et al. Effect of focal lamina cribrosa defect on glaucomatous visual field progression. Ophthalmology 2014;121:1524-1530.
23. Lee EJ, Kim TW. Lamina Cribrosa Reversal after Trabeculectomy and the Rate of Progressive Retinal Nerve Fiber Layer Thinning. Ophthalmology 2015;122:2234-2242.
24. Park SC, Hsu AT, Su D, et al. Factors associated with focal lamina cribrosa defects in glaucoma. Invest Ophthalmol Vis Sci 2013;54:8401-8407.
25. You JY, Park SC, Su D, et al. Focal lamina cribrosa defects associated with glaucomatous rim thinning and acquired pits. JAMA Ophthalmol 2013;131:314-320.

26. Lee EJ, Kim TW, Kim M, et al. Recent structural alteration of the peripheral lamina cribrosa near the location of disc hemorrhage in glaucoma. Invest Ophthalmol Vis Sci 2014;55:2805-2815.
27. Lee EJ, Kim TW, Kim M, Kim H. Influence of lamina cribrosa thickness and depth on the rate of progressive retinal nerve fiber layer thinning. Ophthalmology 2015;122:721-729.
28. Wu Z, Xu G, Weinreb RN, Yu M, Leung CK. Optic Nerve Head Deformation in Glaucoma: A Prospective Analysis of Optic Nerve Head Surface and Lamina Cribrosa Surface Displacement. Ophthalmology 2015;122:1317-1329.
29. Quigley HA, Dunkelberger GR, Green WR. Retinal ganglion cell atrophy correlated with automated perimetry in human eyes with glaucoma. Am J Ophthalmol 1989;107:453-464.
30. Kerrigan-Baumrind LA, Quigley HA, Pease ME, et al. Number of ganglion cells in glaucoma eyes compared with threshold visual field tests in the same persons, Invest Ophthalmol Vis Sci 2000;41:741-748.
31. Medeiros FA, Alencar LM, Zangwill LM, et al. Prediction of functional loss in glaucoma from progressive optic disc damage. Arch Ophthalmol 2009;127:1250-1256.
32. Chauhan BC, Nicolela MT, Artes PH. Incidence and rates of visual field progression after longitudinally measured optic disc change in glaucoma. Ophthalmology 2009;116:2110-2118.
33. Yu M, Lin C, Weinreb RN, et al. Risk of Visual Field Progression in Glaucoma Patients with Progressive Retinal Nerve Fiber Layer Thinning: A 5-Year Prospective Study. Ophthalmology 2016. (In press)
34. Keltner JL, Johnson CA, Anderson DR, et al.; Ocular Hypertension Treatment Study Group. The association between glaucomatous visual fields and optic nerve head features in the Ocular Hypertension Treatment Study. Ophthalmology 2006;113:1603-1612.
35. O'Neill EC, Danesh-Meyer HV, Kong GX, et al. Optic disc evaluation in optic neuropathies: the optic disc assessment project. Ophthalmology 2011;118:964-970.
36. Nonglaucomatous excavation of the optic disc. Trobe JD, Glaser JS, Cassady J, Herschler J, Anderson DR. Arch Ophthalmol 1980;98:1046-1050.
37. Greenfield DS, Siatkowski RM, Glaser JS, Schatz NJ, Parrish RK 2nd. The cupped disc. Who needs neuroimaging? Ophthalmology 1998;105:1866-1874.
38. Wu H, de Boer JF, Chen TC. Diagnostic capability of spectral-domain optical coherence tomography for glaucoma. Am J Ophthalmol 2012;153:815-826 e812.
39. Yang Z, Tatham AJ, Zangwill LM, et al. Diagnostic ability of retinal nerve fiber layer imaging by swept-source optical coherence tomography in glaucoma. Am J Ophthalmol 2015;159:193-201.
40. Silverman AL, Hammel N, Khachatryan N, et al. Diagnostic Accuracy of the Spectralis and Cirrus Reference Databases in Differentiating between Healthy and Early Glaucoma Eyes. Ophthalmology 2016;123:408-414.
41. Leung CK, Lam S, Weinreb RN, et al. Retinal nerve fiber layer imaging with spectral-domain optical coherence tomography: analysis of the retinal nerve fiber layer map for glaucoma detection. Ophthalmology 2010;117:1684-1691.
42. Cheung CY, Chan N, Leung CK. Retinal Nerve Fiber Layer Imaging with Spectral-Domain Optical Coherence Tomography: Impact of Signal Strength on Analysis of the RNFL Map. Asia-Pacific J Ophthalmol 2012;1:19-23.
43. Rao HL, Addepalli UK, Yadav RK, et al. Effect of scan quality on diagnostic accuracy of spectral-domain optical coherence tomography in glaucoma. Am J Ophthalmol 2014;157:719-727 e711.

44. Asrani S, Essaid L, Alder BD, Santiago-Turla C. Artifacts in spectral-domain optical coherence tomography measurements in glaucoma. JAMA Ophthalmol 2014;132:396-402.
45. Lee EJ, Kim TW, Kim M, Choi YJ. Peripapillary retinoschisis in glaucomatous eyes. PloS one 2014;9:e90129.
46. Hwang YH, Kim YY, Kim HK, Sohn YH. Effect of peripapillary retinoschisis on retinal nerve fibre layer thickness measurement in glaucomatous eyes. Brit J Ophthalmol 2014;98:669-674.
47. Hwang YH, Kim YY. Effect of peripapillary vitreous opacity on retinal nerve fiber layer thickness measurement using optical coherence tomography. Arch Ophthalmol 2012;130:789-792.
48. Hwang YH, Kim MK, Kim DW. Segmentation Errors in Macular Ganglion Cell Analysis as Determined by Optical Coherence Tomography. Ophthalmology 2016;123(5):950-958.
49. Gabriele ML, Ishikawa H, Wollstein G, et al. Optical coherence tomography scan circle location and mean retinal nerve fiber layer measurement variability. Invest Ophthalmol Vis Sci 2008;49:2315-2321.
50. Cheung CY, Yiu CK, Weinreb RN, et al. Effects of scan circle displacement in optical coherence tomography retinal nerve fibre layer thickness measurement: a RNFL modelling study. Eye 2009;23:1436-1441.
51. Hwang YH, Lee JY, Kim YY. The effect of head tilt on the measurements of retinal nerve fibre layer and macular thickness by spectral-domain optical coherence tomography. Brit J Ophthalmol 2011;95:1547-1551.
52. Leung CK, Choi N, Weinreb RN, et al. Retinal nerve fiber layer imaging with spectral-domain optical coherence tomography: pattern of RNFL defects in glaucoma. Ophthalmology 2010;117:2337-2344.
53. Shin JW, Uhm KB, Lee WJ, Kim YJ. Diagnostic ability of retinal nerve fiber layer maps to detect localized retinal nerve fiber layer defects. Eye (Lond) 2013;27:1022-1031.
54. Xu J, Ishikawa H, Wollstein G, et al. Three-dimensional spectral-domain optical coherence tomography data analysis for glaucoma detection. PLoS One 2013;8:e55476.
55. Raza AS, Zhang X, De Moraes CG, et al. Improving glaucoma detection using spatially correspondent clusters of damage and by combining standard automated perimetry and optical coherence tomography. Invest Ophthalmol Vis Sci 2014;55:612-624.
56. Almobarak FA, O'Leary N, Reis AS, et al. Automated segmentation of optic nerve head structures with optical coherence tomography. Invest Ophthalmol Vis Sci 2014;55:1161-1168.
57. Chauhan BC, O'Leary N, Almobarak FA, et al. Enhanced detection of open-angle glaucoma with an anatomically accurate optical coherence tomography-derived neuroretinal rim parameter. Ophthalmology 2013;120:535-543.
58. He L, Ren R, Yang H, et al. Anatomic vs. acquired image frame discordance in spectral domain optical coherence tomography minimum rim measurements. PLoS One 2014;9:e92225.
59. Danthurebandara VM, Sharpe GP, Hutchison DM, et al. Enhanced structure-function relationship in glaucoma with an anatomically and geometrically accurate neuroretinal rim measurement. Invest Ophthalmol Vis Sci 2015;56:98-105.
60. Gardiner SK, Boey PY, Yang H, et al. Structural Measurements for Monitoring Change in Glaucoma: Comparing Retinal Nerve Fiber Layer Thickness With Minimum Rim Width and Area. Invest Ophthalmol Vis Sci 2015;56:6886-6891.
61. Gardiner SK, Ren R, Yang H, et al. A method to estimate the amount of neuroretinal rim tissue in glaucoma: comparison with current methods for measuring rim area. Am J Ophthalmol 2014;157:540-549 e541-542.

62. Danthurebandara VM, Vianna JR, Sharpe GP, et al. Diagnostic Accuracy of Glaucoma With Sector-Based and a New Total Profile-Based Analysis of Neuroretinal Rim and Retinal Nerve Fiber Layer Thickness. Invest Ophthalmol Vis Sci 2016;57:181-187.
63. Malik R, Belliveau AC, Sharpe GP, et al. Diagnostic Accuracy of Optical Coherence Tomography and Scanning Laser Tomography for Identifying Glaucoma in Myopic Eyes. Ophthalmology 2016;123(6):1181-1190.
64. Dai Y, Jonas JB, Huang H, Wang M, Sun X. Microstructure of parapapillary atrophy: beta zone and gamma zone. Invest Ophthalmol Vis Sci 2013;54:2013-2018.
65. Choi JA, Kim JS, Park HY, Park H, Park CK. The foveal position relative to the optic disc and the retinal nerve fiber layer thickness profile in myopia. Invest Ophthalmol Vis Sci 2014;55:1419-1426.
66. Chauhan BC, Danthurebandara VM, Sharpe GP, et al. Bruch's Membrane Opening Minimum Rim Width and Retinal Nerve Fiber Layer Thickness in a Normal White Population: A Multicenter Study. Ophthalmology 2015;122:1786-1794.
67. Amini N, Nowroozizadeh S, Cirineo N, et al. Influence of the disc-fovea angle on limits of RNFL variability and glaucoma discrimination. Invest Ophthalmol Vis Sci 2014;55:7332-7342.
68. Hood DC, Raza AS, de Moraes CG, Liebmann JM, Ritch R. Glaucomatous damage of the macula. Prog Retin Eye Res 2013;32:1-21.
69. Hood DC, Raza AS. On improving the use of OCT imaging for detecting glaucomatous damage. Br J Ophthalmol 2014;98(Suppl 2):ii1-9.
70. Hood DC, Slobodnick A, Raza AS, de Moraes CG, Teng CC, Ritch R. Early glaucoma involves both deep local, and shallow widespread, retinal nerve fiber damage of the macular region. Invest Ophthalmol Vis Sci 2014;55:632-649.
71. Oddone F, Lucenteforte E, Michelessi M, et al. Macular versus Retinal Nerve Fiber Layer Parameters for Diagnosing Manifest Glaucoma: A Systematic Review of Diagnostic Accuracy Studies. Ophthalmology 2016;123(5):939-949.
72. Wang DL, Raza AS, de Moraes CG, et al. Central Glaucomatous Damage of the Macula Can Be Overlooked by Conventional OCT Retinal Nerve Fiber Layer Thickness Analyses. Transl Vis Sci Technol 2015;4:4.
73. Hood DC, Xin D, Wang D, et al. A Region-of-Interest Approach for Detecting Progression of Glaucomatous Damage With Optical Coherence Tomography. JAMA Ophthalmol 2015;133:1438-1444.
74. Loewen NA, Zhang X, Tan O, et al. Advanced Imaging for Glaucoma Study G. Combining measurements from three anatomical areas for glaucoma diagnosis using Fourier-domain optical coherence tomography. Br J Ophthalmol 2015;99:1224-1229.
75. Realini T, Zangwill LM, Flanagan JG, et al. Normative Databases for Imaging Instrumentation. J Glaucoma 2015;24:480-483.
76. Tatham AJ, Miki A, Weinreb RN, Zangwill LM, Medeiros FA. Defects of the lamina cribrosa in eyes with localized retinal nerve fiber layer loss. Ophthalmology 2014;121:110-118.
77. Weinreb RN, Aung T, Medeiros FA. The pathophysiology and treatment of glaucoma: a review. JAMA 2014;311:1901-1911.
78. Fechtner RD, Weinreb RN. Mechanisms of optic nerve damage in primary open angle glaucoma. Surv Ophthalmol 1994;39:23-42.
79. Anderson DR. Ultrastructure of human and monkey lamina cribrosa and optic nerve head. Arch Ophthalmol 1969;82:800-814.
80. Wilczek M. The lamina cribrosa and its nature. Br J Ophthalmol 1947;31:551-565.

81. You JY, Park SC, Su D, et al. Focal Lamina Cribrosa Defects Associated With Glaucomatous Rim Thinning and Acquired Pits. JAMA Ophthalmology 2013;131:314.
82. Kiumehr S, Park SC, Syril D, et al. In vivo evaluation of focal lamina cribrosa defects in glaucoma. Arch Ophthalmol 2012;130:552-559.
83. Kim TW, Kagemann L, Girard MJ, et al. Imaging of the lamina cribrosa in glaucoma: perspectives of pathogenesis and clinical applications. Curr Eye Res 2013;38:903-909.
84. Burgoyne CF, Downs JC, Bellezza AJ, Suh JK, Hart RT. The optic nerve head as a biomechanical structure: a new paradigm for understanding the role of IOP-related stress and strain in the pathophysiology of glaucomatous optic nerve head damage. Prog Retin Eye Res 2005;24:39-73.
85. Chung HS, Sung KR, Lee KS, Lee JR, Kim S. Relationship between the lamina cribrosa, outer retina, and choroidal thickness as assessed using spectral domain optical coherence tomography. Korean J Ophthalmol 2014;28:234-240.
86. Genovese K, Casaletto L, Lee YU, Humphrey JD. Panoramic stereo DIC-based strain measurement on submerged objects. In: Proulx T (Ed.), Optical measurements, Modeling and Metrology, vol. 5, pp. 257-263. New York: Springer 2011.
87. Lee EJ, Kim TW, Weinreb RN, rk KH, Kim SH, Kim DM. Three-dimensional evaluation of the lamina cribrosa using spectral-domain optical coherence tomography in glaucoma. Invest Ophthalmol Vis Sci 2012;53:198-204.
88. Mansouri K, Nuyen B, R NW. Improved visualization of deep ocular structures in glaucoma using high penetration optical coherence tomography. Expert Rev Med Devices 2013;10:621-628.
89. Mari JM, Strouthidis NG, Park SC, Girard MJ. Enhancement of lamina cribrosa visibility in optical coherence tomography images using adaptive compensation. Invest Ophthalmol Vis Sci 2013;54:2238-2247.
90. Miki A, Ikuno Y, Jo Y, Nishida K. Comparison of enhanced depth imaging and high-penetration optical coherence tomography for imaging deep optic nerve head and parapapillary structures. Clin Ophthalmol 2013;7:1995-2001.
91. Park SC, Ritch R. High resolution in vivo imaging of the lamina cribrosa. Saudi J Ophthalmol 2011;25:363-372.
92. Kim YK, Park KH. Lamina cribrosa defects in eyes with glaucomatous disc haemorrhage. Acta Ophthalmologica 2015;n/a-n/a.
93. Lee EJ, Kim TW, Weinreb RN. Reversal of lamina cribrosa displacement and thickness after trabeculectomy in glaucoma. Ophthalmology 2012;119:1359-1366.
94. Rhodes LA, Huisingh C, Johnstone J, Fazio M, Smith B, Clark M, Downs JC, Owsley C, Girard MJ, Mari JM, Girkin C. Variation of laminar depth in normal eyes with age and race. Invest Ophthalmol Vis Sci 2014;55:8123-8133.
95. Furlanetto RL, Park SC, Damle UJ, Sieminski SF, Kung Y, Siegal N, Liebmann JM, Ritch R. Posterior displacement of the lamina cribrosa in glaucoma: in vivo interindividual and intereye comparisons. Invest Ophthalmol Vis Sci 2013;54:4836-4842.
96. Ren R, Yang H, Gardiner SK, Fortune B, Hardin C, Demirel S, Burgoyne CF. Anterior lamina cribrosa surface depth, age, and visual field sensitivity in the Portland Progression Project. Invest Ophthalmol Vis Sci 2014;55:1531-1539.
97. Belghith A, Bowd C, Medeiros FA, Weinreb RN, Zangwill LM. Automated Segmentation of Anterior Lamina Cribrosa Surface: How the Lamina Cribrosa Responds to Intraocular Pressure Change in Glaucoma Eyes. IEEE International Symposium on Biomedical Imaging ISBI. New York; 2015:222-225.

98. Xu G, Weinreb RN, Leung CK. Optic nerve head deformation in glaucoma: the temporal relationship between optic nerve head surface depression and retinal nerve fiber layer thinning. Ophthalmology 2014;121:2362-2370.
99. Leung CK, Mohamed S, Leung KS, et al. Retinal nerve fiber layer measurements in myopia: An optical coherence tomography study. Invest Ophthalmol Vis Sci. 2006;47:5171-6.
100. Vernon SA, Rotchford AP, Negi A, et al. Peripapillary retinal nerve fibre layer thickness in highly myopic Caucasians as measured by Stratus optical coherence tomography. Br J Ophthalmol. 2008;92:1076-80.
101. Aref AA, Sayyad FE, Mwanza JC, et al. Diagnostic specificities of retinal nerve fiber layer, optic nerve head, and macular ganglion cell-inner plexiform layer measurements in myopic eyes. J Glaucoma. 2014;23:487-493.
102. Leal-Fonseca M, Rebolleda G, Oblanca N,et al. A comparison of false positives in retinal nerve fiber layer, optic nerve head and macular ganglion cell-inner plexiform layer from two spectral-domain optical coherence tomography devices. Graefes Arch Clin Exp Ophthalmol. 2014;252:321-330.
103. Yamashita T, Kii Y, Tanaka M, et al. Relationship between supernormal sectors of retinal nerve fibre layer and axial length in normal eyes. Acta Ophthalmol. 2014;92:e481-487.
104. Kim KE, Jeoung JW, Park KH, et al. Diagnostic classification of macular ganglion cell and retinal nerve fiber layer analysis: differentiation of false-positives from glaucoma. Ophthalmology. 2015;122:502-510.
105. Qiu KL, Zhang MZ, Leung CK, et al. Diagnostic classification of retinal nerve fiber layer measurement in myopic eyes: a comparison between time-domain and spectral-domain optical coherence tomography. Am J Ophthalmol. 2011;152:646-653.
106. Leung CK, Yu M, Weinreb RN, et al. Retinal Nerve Fiber Layer Imaging with Spectral-Domain Optical Coherence Tomography: Interpreting the RNFL Maps in Healthy Myopic Eyes. Invest Ophthalmol Vis Sci. 2012;53:7194-200.
107. Biswas S, Lin C, Leung CK. Evaluation of a Myopic Normative Database for Analysis of Retinal Nerve Fiber Layer Thickness. JAMA Ophthalmol. 2016 In press.
108. Sigal IA, Flanagan JG, Ethier CR. Factors influencing optic nerve head biomechanics. Invest Ophthalmol Vis Sci 2005;46: 4189-4199
109. Sigal IA, Yang H, Roberts MD, Grimm JL, Burgoyne CF, Demirel S, Downs JC. IOP-induced lamina cribrosa deformation and scleral canal expansion: independent or related? Invest Ophthalmol Vis Sci. 2011;52:9023-9032
110. Quigley H, Anderson DR. The dynamics and location of axonal transport blockade by acute intraocular pressure elevation in primate optic nerve. Invest Ophthalmol. 1976;15:606-616.
111. Quigley HA, Anderson DR. Distribution of axonal transport blockade by acute intraocular pressure elevation in the primate optic nerve head. Invest Ophthalmol Vis Sci. 1977;16:640-644.
112. Quigley HA, Addicks EM. Chronic experimental glaucoma in primates. II. Effect of extended intraocular pressure elevation on optic nerve head and axonal transport. Invest Ophthalmol Vis Sci. 1980;19:137-152.
113. Geijer C, Bill A. Effects of raised intraocular pressure on retinal, prelaminar, laminar, and retrolaminar optic nerve blood flow in monkeys. Invest Ophthalmol Vis Sci. 1979 Oct;18(10):1030-1042.
114. Radius RL. Optic nerve fast axonal transport abnormalities in primates. Occurrence after short posterior ciliary artery occlusion. Arch Ophthalmol. 1980;98:2018-2022.

115. Downs JC, Yang H, Girkin C, Sakata L, Bellezza A, Thompson H, Burgoyne CF. Three-dimensional histomorphometry of the normal and early glaucomatous monkey optic nerve head: neural canal and subarachnoid space architecture. Invest Ophthalmol Vis Sci. 2007;48:3195-3208.

116. Yang H, Downs JC, Girkin C, Sakata L, Bellezza A, Thompson H, Burgoyne CF. 3-D histomorphometry of the normal and early glaucomatous monkey optic nerve head: lamina cribrosa and peripapillary scleral position and thickness. Invest Ophthalmol Vis Sci. 2007;48:4597-4607.

117. Yang H, Williams G, Downs JC, Sigal IA, Roberts MD, Thompson H, Burgoyne CF. Posterior (outward) migration of the lamina cribrosa and early cupping in monkey experimental glaucoma. Invest Ophthalmol Vis Sci. 2011;52:7109-7121.

118. Downs JC, Suh JK, Thomas KA, Bellezza AJ, Burgoyne CF, Hart RT. Viscoelastic characterization of peripapillary sclera: material properties by quadrant in rabbit and monkey eyes. J Biomech Eng. 2003;125:124-131.

119. Girard MJ, Suh JK, Bottlang M, Burgoyne CF, Downs JC. Biomechanical changes in the sclera of monkey eyes exposed to chronic IOP elevations. Invest Ophthalmol Vis Sci. 2011;52:5656-5669.

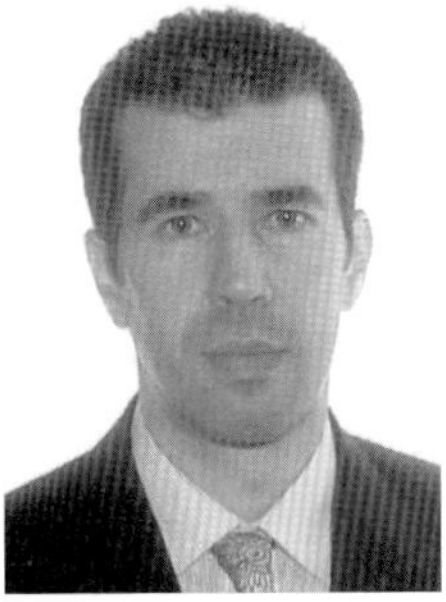
David Garway-Heath

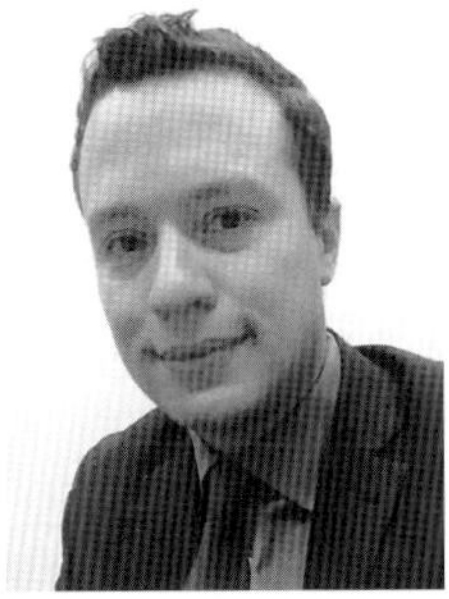
Gustavo De Moraes

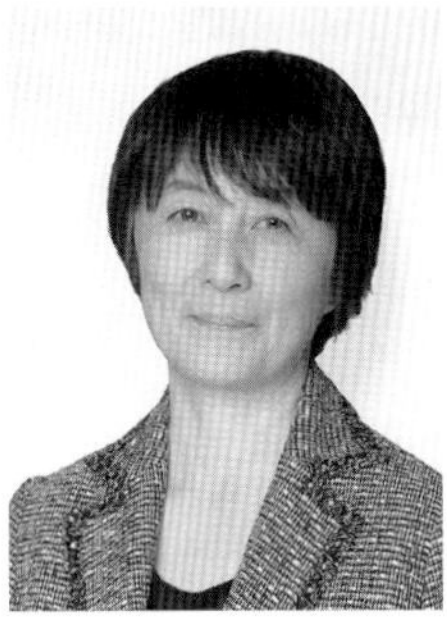
Aiko Iwase

2. VISION FUNCTION

Section leader: David Garway-Heath
Section co-leaders: Gustavo De Moraes, Aiko Iwase
Contributors: Andrew Anderson, Makoto Araie, Ryo Asaoka, Augusto Azuara-Blanco, Christopher Bowd, Paolo Brusini, Joseph Caprioli, Jack Cioffi, David Crabb, Barbara C. Venkel, Robert Fechtner, Brad Fortune, Paul Foster, Stuart Gardiner, Fransicso Javier Goni, David Henson, Donald Hood, Chris A. Johnson, Chota Matsumoto, Allison Maree Mckendrick, Andrew McNaught, Jonathan Myers, Pradeep Ramulu, Remo Susanna Jr, Michael Wall

Consensus statements

1. Functional testing is essential for the evaluation, staging and monitoring of glaucoma.
   Comment: Standard automated perimetry (SAP) is the reference standard for all functional testing.
2. Clinical decisions should be made based on reliable visual field tests.
   Comments: Visual field defects should be reproducible and/or should be consistent with the location of the optic nerve defects.
   The most important reliability criterion is the false positive rate.
3. In the presence of glaucomatous optic neuropathy, a Glaucoma Hemifield Test (GHT) 'outside normal limits' in a reliable visual field indicates that glaucomatous visual field loss is present.
   Comment: For instruments not calculating a GHT, an abnormal ($P < 5\%$) pattern standard deviation (PSD) or square-root-loss variance (sLV) likely have similar diagnostic value.
4. When glaucomatous optic neuropathy (GON) is suspected, a GHT criterion of 'outside normal limits' or 'borderline' in a reliable visual field increases the probability that an eye has glaucoma.
   Comment: The level of probability for glaucoma depends on the presence and magnitude of other risk factors for glaucoma (such as raised intraocular pressure) and the quality of evidence that there is no GON.

Diagnosis of Primary Open Angle Glaucoma, pp 21-89
Edited by Robert N. Weinreb, David Garway-Heath, Christopher Leung, Felipe Medeiros, Jeffrey Liebmann

5. Before a visual field defect can be confirmed as glaucomatous, retinal and non-glaucomatous optic disc conditions should be excluded by a careful examination of the retina and optic disc.
   Comment: If the pattern of visual field loss suggests a neurological origin, or if there is incongruity between the pattern of visual field loss and optic disc and retinal nerve fiber layer appearance, then further investigation is warranted (*e.g.*, color vision testing, neuroimaging).
6. Standard white-on-white automated perimetry (SAP), with a fixed testing matrix covering at least the central 24 degrees, is preferred for the diagnosis of glaucomatous visual field loss.
   Comments: Goldmann size III stimuli are conventionally used in most automated perimeters in clinical practice for glaucoma diagnosis.
   For more severe cases size V, increases the dynamic range and reduces variability of test results.
   Using the 10-2 strategy, in addition to the conventional 24-2 Humphrey grid, can improve the detection of central functional loss.
7. Threshold algorithms are preferred over supra-threshold algorithms for glaucoma diagnosis.
   Comment: Supra-threshold algorithms can be helpful in cases of unreliable results from threshold testing algorithms.
8. Neither short-wavelength automated perimetry (SWAP) nor frequency doubling technology (FDT) perimetry have superior diagnostic precision to SAP.
   Comments: Patients should be followed consistently with same visual function test and ideally one with statistical support for recognizing change.
   The more diagnostic tests that are performed, the more likely it is that one will be 'outside normal limits', therefore increasing the number of false positive results.
9. Patients who are at risk for glaucoma and have normal standard automated perimetry (SAP) should have their visual function monitored to detect deterioration and hence establish a glaucoma diagnosis.
   Comment: The earliest evidence for glaucoma may be functional or structural. Therefore, both should be measured to ensure that the onset of glaucoma damage is not overlooked.
10. Deterioration may be first detected by the glaucoma hemifield test (GHT) (or summary parameters) or by trend analysis of measurements over time. Which analysis is most sensitive varies between patients and so both should be done.

Comments: Progressive functional loss identified by SAP may be a generalized reduction in visual field sensitivity alone, or focal loss alone, or a combination of both.

If trend analysis indicates a change in VFI, MD or mean defect, then one needs to exclude media opacity (*e.g.*, cataract).

11. There only is weak evidence for the use of functional measurements other than SAP to detect the earliest signs of deterioration.
12. There is a limited role for ERG testing in the routine diagnosis and management of glaucoma.

    Comment: PERG and PhNR testing are not substitutes for standard automated perimetry (SAP), nor are they substitutes for optical coherence tomography (OCT) imaging.
13. The classification of glaucomatous functional damage in stages of increasing severity is a useful tool in the management of patients affected with chronic glaucoma.

    Comment: Staging provides a summary metric of disease severity which may guide treatment decisions.
14. While staging systems may be clinically useful, no current staging system shows all the information present in a visual field printout.

    Comment: For instance, staging systems do not identify the location of damage.
15. POAG-related functional impairment affects patients' ability to perform daily activities and also their well-being (vision-related quality of life). Worse vision-related quality of life is associated with greater severity of the disease.

    Comment: Vision-related quality of life may be assessed with questionnaires, by performance tasks (*e.g.*, reading), event monitoring (*e.g.*, falls) and measures of behavior (*e.g.*, GPS trackers).
16. Understanding how glaucoma and glaucoma treatment affects patients' quality of life, and how this varies across the severity continuum, can have practical value in the clinic. It can inform treatment choices and communication to patients of the implications of disease worsening.
17. The impact of glaucomatous visual field loss on vision-related function and quality of life depends on the location of the defect in the field of vision and the task involved.

    Comment: risk of falling, eye-hand coordination and mobility may be most affected by loss in the inferior hemifield, whereas reading may be more affected by superior hemifield loss.

18. Aspects of glaucoma other than visual field loss, such as reduced central contrast sensitivity and acuity (in more advanced disease), may affect vision-related function and quality of life.
    Comment: Contrast sensitivity is more strongly associated with specific aspects of reading performance than visual field measures.

2.1. Diagnosis based on Standard Automated Perimetry SAP 24-2

Andrew Anderson, Ryo Asaoka, Paolo Brusini, Joseph Caprioli, Jack Cioffi, Stuart Gardiner

2.1.1. Diagnostic criteria in the presence of suspected (equivocal) glaucomatous optic neuropathy (GON)

A variety of diagnostic criteria has been used in the literature for SAP visual fields, and although some strategies are more common than others, no clear consensus exists as to the best criterion. The quality of the studies assessing the performance of diagnostic methods is also variable. Of the five studies assessing the performance of SAP that met the inclusion criteria of a review by Burr *et al.*,[1] only one study of the five met their criteria for higher quality studies (being Robin *et al.*[2]). Scoring systems, appropriate for research purposes, to establish whether a visual field defect is present, such as the Advanced Glaucoma Intervention Study (AGIS) system, are likely too complex and time consuming for use in busy clinical environments (see section on Scoring systems). The use of simplified methods is therefore more appropriate.

Attempts to directly compare sensitivity and specificity values for SAP diagnostic criteria reported in the literature is complicated by the fact that different studies use different inclusion and exclusion criteria for study participants. In particular, the use of criteria that tightly define glaucomatous and control groups, and excludes participants failing to meet the criteria for either group, tend to exaggerate the difference between groups and so elevate sensitivity and specificity estimates;[3] the magnitude of this elevation is difficult to assess. In particular, clinical studies typically exclude participants with cataract, other diseases that may affect visual function, and may have very few participants over 80 years old, yet it is these very people who make up a considerable proportion of patients seen clinically. The generalizability to clinical practice of such studies is, therefore, limited. However, assessing the relative performance of methods within a study is still informative. Katz *et al.*[4] performed such an assessment, and obtained the following results for those methods that do not require additional calculation when using the HFA perimeter (Table 1). For comparison, results obtained using the AGIS classification for identifying a visual field defect (which seeks clusters of depressed points in three subdivisions of the visual field) are also included.

Overall, this analysis found little difference between methods, aside from a trade-off between sensitivity and specificity. Combination of methods (*e.g.*, abnormal CPSD or GHT) only slightly increased sensitivity, at the expense of a lowered specificity. Of note is that the CPSD is no longer a feature of the analysis provided by SITA visual fields, and that confidence intervals for their sensitivity/specificity values were not provided. For comparison, Robin *et al.*[2] performed a community-based assessment of glaucoma detection and found the sensitivity and specificity for glaucoma identification with AGIS scores (score $\geq$ 1) of 90 and 58, respectively, giving a positive predictive value of 14% and a negative predictive value of 99%. This somewhat lower performance than that seen in Table 1 likely reflects that the well-defined glaucoma and control groups in Katz *et al.*[4] may have resulted in an overestimation of diagnostic performance. That Katz *et al.*[4] used the presence of a visual field defect on manual perimetry in their definition of glaucoma likely also overestimated the absolute diagnostic performance of perimetry for detecting glaucoma.

No single index can reliably detect all glaucomatous defects. Asaoka *et al.*[5] compared visual fields from pre-perimetric GON eyes (*i.e.*, not satisfying the commonly used Anderson-Patella criteria for visual field loss) to healthy eyes and found significant sensitivity loss was present, particularly in the nasal step and Bjerrum areas. This suggests it is useful to carefully evaluate the visual field test result, considering the structural damage and how it likely relates to functional

Table 1. Comparison of different criteria for diagnosing visual field defects on the Humphrey Field Analyzer, taken from Katz *et al.*[4] Only the situation when visual field results are considered reliable is considered.

Method	**Sensitivity**	**Specificity**
MD, P < 5%	81	92
MD, P < 1%	70	98
CPSD, P < 5%	96	90
CPSD, P < 1%	79	97
GHT ('outside normal limits' only)	97	86
GHT ('outside normal limits' or borderline)	99	84
AGIS	96	78

loss, even in pre-perimetric eyes. Whilst such assessment is likely appropriate when performed by highly trained glaucoma specialists, it is not clear that such an assessment will result in a diagnostic performance better – or even comparable to – that seen by simple statistical indices when performed by eye care clinicians without specialist glaucoma training.

Recommendation

Overall, when using the HFA, the simplicity of the GHT – both in terms of its plain language reporting, and that it requires no calculation – recommends its use as the primary diagnostic index for the presence of a glaucomatous visual field defect in clinical settings. Where GON is suspected, a **GHT criterion of 'outside normal limits' or 'borderline'** is recommended **for providing additional evidence that a person has glaucoma,**[6] with 'outside normal limits' providing stronger evidence than 'borderline'. This criterion is appropriate to maximize sensitivity rather than specificity, although it is noted that only limited differences were found by Katz *et al.*[4] between GHT criteria (outside normal limits ± borderline). Where GON is suspected, only a **GHT criterion of 'outside normal limits'** is recommended **for establishing that a visual field defect is present** (*i.e.*, a 'borderline' result is insufficient).

In all circumstances it should first be established that the visual field agrees with additional information. This agreement should be:

i. that any loss in the visual field is in the hemifield predicted by the GON or, when this is not the case;
ii. that on a subsequent visual field examination, the GHT classification is confirmed and any loss is in the same hemifield as the original visual field.

The above criteria should only be applied to those visual fields judged to be reliable, which includes an examination of maps of deviation from normal so that any irregularities or artifacts can be assessed.

Before a visual field defect can be confirmed as glaucomatous, retinal conditions should be excluded by a careful examination of the fundus and optic nerve conditions (*e.g.*, disc drusen) should be excluded by a careful examination of the optic disc. If the pattern of visual field loss suggests a neurological origin, or if there is incongruity between the pattern of visual field loss and optic disc and retinal nerve fiber layer appearance, then further investigation is warranted (*e.g.*, color vision testing, neuroimaging).

For instruments where the GHT or its equivalent is not calculated, an abnormal ($p < 5\%$) PSD or equivalent (*e.g.*, square root of the loss variance, sLV) will likely give a similar diagnostic performance based on the findings of Katz *et al.*[4] using the related index CPSD. As above, visual fields must be reliable and defects show appropriate agreement with other information.

No single index can detect all glaucomatous visual field defects. Whilst glaucoma specialists performing a visual evaluation of a visual field test result may have a diagnostic accuracy that exceeds visual field statistical indices, including that of the GHT recommended above, there is insufficient evidence to establish that this is the case for eye care clinicians without specialist glaucoma training.

2.1.2. Diagnostic criteria in the absence of glaucomatous optic neuropathy (GON)

Perimetric assessment is important for the diagnosis of glaucoma, even in the absence of suspected GON. For example, in a population screening in Australia[7] 49% of those with previously undiagnosed glaucoma had seen an optometrist or ophthalmologist in the previous year. Almost all previously undiagnosed cases (97%) had visual field defects. A statistically significant factor separating previously diagnosed and previously undiagnosed glaucoma was the presence of a visual field defect, suggesting a bias towards the use of structural information in clinical diagnosis. Given that perimetry is typically performed if clinically indicated and that such indications are commonly based on assessments of structure (*e.g.*, suspicious optic nerve heads), this bias likely reflects, at least in part, the way in which testing for glaucoma is usually performed, rather than indicating that structure necessarily provides superior information for diagnosis. Such a bias towards structure assessment may also exist in the selection of participants for research studies evaluating glaucoma diagnostic tests; although a structure reference is appropriate when evaluating the *relative* performance of various perimetric tests, the *absolute* performance of perimetric tests is likely underestimated because glaucomatous eyes with abnormal perimetry, but structural measures within the normal range, are not included.

Recommendation

When GON is **not** suspected, only a **GHT criterion of 'outside normal limits'** is recommended **for providing evidence that a person has glaucoma** (*i.e.*, a classification of 'borderline' is insufficient), in order to minimize false-positive calls[4]). Similarly, only a **GHT criterion of 'outside normal limits'** is recommended

for establishing that a visual field defect is present. The level of probability for glaucoma depends on the presence and magnitude of other risk factors for glaucoma (such as raised intraocular pressure) and the quality of evidence that there is no GON.

All other recommendations are as given above for when GON is suspected, including those regarding the need for visual field results to be both reliable and in agreement with other information. As GON is not suspected, agreement with optic nerve assessment findings is not possible. Therefore, performance of a subsequent visual field is mandatory, with agreement established by ensuring the GHT classification is confirmed and that any loss is in the same hemifield as in the original visual field.

2.1.3. Criteria in the presence of clinically certain GON

When the presence of GON is clinically certain, it is likely that most clinicians will have already made a diagnosis of glaucoma on this finding alone. Consequently, criteria regarding the presence or absence of a visual field defect are not primarily for the diagnosis of glaucoma per se but for whether a significant visual field defect accompanies the glaucoma.

Recommendation

When GON is clinically certain, only a **GHT criterion of 'outside normal limits'** is recommended **for establishing that a visual field defect is also present** (*i.e.*, a classification of 'borderline' is insufficient). A GHT of 'borderline' raises the probability that glaucomatous visual field loss is present, with structure/function concordance and repeatable defects resulting in higher probability. All other recommendations are as given above for when GON is suspected, including those regarding the need for visual field results to be both reliable and in agreement with other information. This agreement should be:

i. that any loss in the visual field is in the hemifield predicted by the GON or, when this is not the case;
ii. that on a subsequent visual field examination, the GHT classification is confirmed and any loss is in the same hemifield as the original visual field.

2.2. Alternative Standard Automated Perimetry Algorithms

Gustavo de Moraes, Allison Maree Mckendrick

2.2.1. Research Needs

1. Improvements to perimetric test strategies have been proposed based on computer simulation studies, including changes to stimulus test locations and thresholding algorithms. These now need validation in clinical practice with a diversity of patients.
2. The role of customizing visual field test algorithms for individuals (based on their prior results, anatomical features, or disease status) requires further research.
3. The ability to incorporate additional test points in the superior macular region in clinical instrumentation with easy user interface and analysis tools is required to facilitate evaluation.
4. Given the high test-retest variability for locations with marked visual field damage (sensitivity < approximately 15 dB), further assessment of the benefits of attempting to threshold these locations (relative to testing new locations) is required.
5. Further investigation of the pros and cons of varying the size of visual field stimuli with eccentricity is required, in particular with respect to maintaining a constant size relationship with respect to Ricco's area (the stimulus size that limits complete spatial summation for any given location). This work requires consideration of individual differences, including variations to stimulus size in retinal space that arise due variation in axial length (especially in myopia).
6. Current research suggests that the detection of visual field damage may be assisted by changing stimulus size, or test pattern location, and that further benefits could be achieved if such factors varied on an individual patient basis. Such an approach requires novel analytical methods to be developed for the subsequent determination of progression of damage, if the visual field test applied to the patient varies with time.

One of the limitations of standard automated perimetry (SAP) is the increase in variability of test locations as defects become deeper.[8] Some of the existing perimetric testing algorithms are: (1) the Full-Threshold visual field test with 4-2-1 bracketing strategy; (2) the Swedish Interactive Testing Algorithm (SITA)\;,[9] (3) the German Adaptive Thresholding Estimation;[10] and (4) the Zippy Estimation by

Sequential Testing (ZEST).[11] The performance of all these algorithms is limited by the increase in variability with disease worsening, whilst at the same time they need to maintain a short test duration so that the reliability is not compromised by fatigue.[12]

Detailed experiments of the likelihood of responding to particular stimulus intensities at a retinal location (measured with frequency-of-seeing (FOS) curves which are sigmoidal in shape) demonstrate the range of stimulus intensities over which an observer's probability of response shifts from being highly likely to highly unlikely is wider in areas of visual field damage (in other words, predictability of responses to a given stimulus intensity is reduced in areas of visual field with relative scotoma).[13] To illustrate, the following is an abridged description of how the fundamental visual perceptual responses described by the FOS curve slope influence the probability an individual responds to perimetric stimuli and therefore perimetric threshold algorithm performance. Automated perimetry typically uses a 3.5 log unit (35 dB) range of stimulus contrasts to assess function within the visual field. While an eye is being tested, the algorithm will test and retest each location many times, either increasing stimulus intensity (if not seen) or reducing intensity (if seen), with many algorithms (*e.g.*, Full Threshold, or SITA: Carl Zeiss Meditec, Inc.) using a fixed interval (step size), until it converges to the threshold sensitivity. Let us consider two hypothetical locations, one initially tested at 10 dB and another tested at 25 dB. At both of these locations, the patient does not respond (a 'not seen' response). For a location that has a true threshold of 10 dB (with greater variability: standard deviation of the cumulative Gaussian used to describe their sigmoidal FOS of 5 dB), if the stimulus is shown at 10 dB, the subject has a 50% chance of seeing it. If shown 5 dB brighter, at 5 dB (one standard deviation greater than 10 dB), they have about a 68% chance of seeing it. At another, more sensitive, location, with a true threshold of 25 dB (and low variability: a standard deviation of FOS of 1 dB), if the stimulus is shown at 25 dB, the subject has a 50% chance of seeing it. However, if the same 5 dB increment is applied (to at stimulus intensity of 20 dB) the subject now has close to a 100% chance of seeing it. These steps, based upon fixed increments or decrements of sensitivity (*i.e.*, not taking into account the variability in response probability as a function of sensitivity), can be problematic as it increases the time to converge to the threshold sensitivity at that location and increases the chance of erroneous threshold estimates being returned. As an attempt to overcome this challenge, Gardiner proposed a variability-adjusted algorithm.[14] Such an algorithm instead scales the step-size (increment or decrement of intensity for the next stimulus presentation) for each location based on the likely FOS curve standard deviation (variability of response probability). This likely FOS curve is determined from previous descriptions of FOS as a function of perimetric sensitivity,[13] and is estimated on a trial-by-trial basis depending on the subjects response to a given stimulus. In short, as the stimulus intensity increases (because the subject has not seen the stimulus), the step-size of the algorithm also increases to account for increased response variability in areas of visual field damage. Therefore, the algorithm should perform more efficiently when measuring locations with low sensitivities. Added to that, customized algorithms, such as variability-adjusted algorithms, would spend less time testing areas with sensitivities below 15 dB as these areas tend to provide less reliable information.[15]

Another alternative is to modify the stimulus size. Goldmann isopter III-4e is the most widely used stimulus size in automated perimetry and is also used for legal definitions of blindness. It consists of a target of 0.43 degrees of visual angle with a luminance of 318 cd/m^2 (1,000 apostilbs). Perimetric contrast sensitivity is known to increase with stimulus size in both normal and diseased eyes. It has been proposed that use of a size V-4e (1.8 degrees of visual angle) stimulus reduces variability, allowing reliable visual field testing to be performed later into the disease process.[16-18] One reason for this is that test-retest variability is lower in areas with abnormal sensitivity when a size V stimulus is used.[16] Also, size-V stimuli have a greater effective dynamic range than size III and have about twice as many discriminable steps. Regarding the dynamic range, the number of steps from normal to blind in SAP is determined by the test-retest variability and the stimulus brightness range. SAP size III has four discriminable steps for progression with a floor around 15-19 dB, below which the reliability of responses becomes compromised, as previously discussed. Investigators who compared the dynamic ranges of different tests and stimulus sizes found that SAP size V has as many as eight discriminable steps for progression and a floor around 4-8 dB.[18] In other words, once patients progress to very low sensitivities with conventional SAP size III, switching to size V could help monitoring changes for a longer period with sustained reliability.

In another study, the investigators found no evidence that use of a size-V stimulus significantly decreased the lower limit of the reliable stimulus range beyond 15 to 19 dB.[19] However, using a size-V stimulus resulted in a higher sensitivity at the same location. For instance, a test location that reached a sensitivity value of 15 dB with size III may reveal a sensitivity of 20 dB when tested with a size V stimulus. This higher sensitivity means that a location will not reach the lower limit of reliable testing until later in the disease process, resulting in more reliable and less variable estimates of sensitivity at damaged visual field locations.

In an ideal scenario, algorithms should automatically make this modification during testing when an area of very depressed sensitivities is identified (or based on previous test results). The Heidelberg Edge Perimeter (HEP) allows the use of a Goldmann size III target for the 40 dB to 16 dB range, whereas from 15 dB to 0 dB, the stimulus size is increased following the Goldmann equation to give perceptual equivalence. For perimeters which do not employ this algorithm, one alternative approach could be to alternate stimulus sizes between test days. The limitation, however, is that progression analyses can only be done by comparing tests with the same stimulus size; thus, the number of tests available for automated progression analysis would decrease (or the time of follow-up would need to be increased).

Alternatively, Khuu and Kalloniatis[20] attempted to establish Ricco's critical area (Ac) at all visual field testing locations of the 30-2 visual field to identify Goldmann test sizes that are within or outside complete spatial summation By doing so, they suggested that it is possible to systematically determine threshold changes across the visual field locations and further characterize the importance of testing within the area of complete spatial summation in SAP.

Another method to modify testing algorithms is to increase the density of test points based upon eccentricity. Once functional damage threatens or affects the central 10 degrees of the visual field, the 24-2 (or 30-2) grid becomes less able to detect abnormalities and monitor changes. With a 6-degree distance between test locations (and 3 degrees from the horizontal and vertical meridians) the total number of points tested within the central 9 degrees is only 4 (plus the foveal sensitivity). This relatively small visual field area encompasses approximately 30% of the ganglion cells of the entire retina[21] and corresponds to over 60% of the visual cortex.[22] By changing the testing strategy to a 10-2 grid, one can now test 68 test points in the central 10 degrees, each separated by 2 degrees (1 degree from the horizontal and vertical meridians) and thus better assess the presence and progression of paracentral damage (Fig. 1).[23,24]

This relatively poor sampling of the central field would be of little concern if glaucoma did not affect the macular region or, for that matter, if initial glaucomatous damage always occurred outside the central macula region. However, it has been clear for at least 30 years that early, and even initial, macular defects occur in some patients.[25] More recently, it has been shown that among eyes with normal 24-2 hemifields, 16% can actually be classified as abnormal when tested

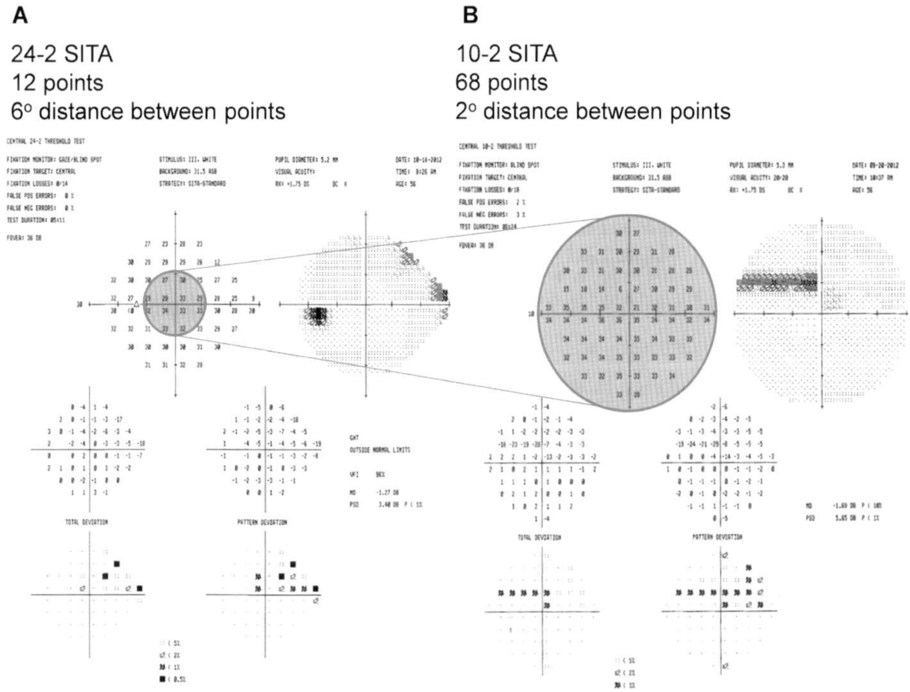

Fig. 1. Comparison of number and distance between tested locations using the A) 24-2 vs. B) 10-2 grids.

with 10-2 algorithm.[23] Thus, 10-2 testing is useful in patents reporting symptoms suggesting central visual field loss, those with structural damage that relates anatomically to the central visual field and those with advanced glaucoma and only central visual field preservation.

Figure 2 depicts an example of how increasing the density of test points with 10-2 improves detection of central damage compared to conventional 24-2 strategy. Despite a total deviation plot with sensitivities between -2 and -5 dB in the central 24-2 field (top figure), a defect seen in the 10-2 (bottom) of the same eye, tested on the same day, falls between the locations tested with the conventional grid (6 degrees apart). This defect would have been overlooked if a 10-2 tests had not been performed and the eye would have been classified as normal or suspect.

Alternatively, it has been shown that adding four points from the 10-2 test pattern to the 24-2 test pattern significantly improved its ability to detect macular defects without employing more test points than a single 10-2 test.[26] In another study, Chen *et al.*[27] employed data collected with a different visual field test

ed automated natural neighbor approach (GOANNA). It begins with a pool of possible test locations (determined in part by the subset of test locations in the 24-2 pattern with highest predictive value for glaucomatous visual field damage described above,[31] and autonomously selects stimulus locations during a visual field test.[33] The locations are chosen so regions surrounding scotoma borders receive increased spatial resolution, without increasing test times. It was shown to improve precision (degree of test-retest variability) and accuracy (difference between the true threshold and the measured threshold) of threshold estimates, while maintaining efficiency (number of presentations) compared with current approaches.

2.3. Alternative Perimetry

Christopher Bowd, Francisco Javier Goñi, Chris A. Johnson, Chota Matsumoto

2.3.1. Research Needs

1. High-quality research studies, with the appropriate reference test for the diagnosis of glaucoma, are required to evaluate the relative diagnostic precision and accuracy of perimetry tests.
   Comment: a structural reference standard, or evidence of progressive damage, is required for perimetry test comparisons.
2. All perimetry tests exhibit marked between-subject and test-retest variability; studies evaluating alternative perimetry should address the signal-to-noise ratio of the tests relative to SAP.

2.3.2. Background

The human eye is able to discriminate certain features associated with light perception including luminosity, contrast and color, as well as dynamic characteristics such as spatial and temporal changes. Glaucoma may affect any or all of these at the different stages of the disease. The visual field can be examined with various methods to test different aspects of visual function. Currently, the most widely used technique is Standard Automated Perimetry (SAP), but other methods have been described, mainly for early glaucoma diagnosis, and are referred to as non-conventional or Alternative Perimetry (AP). These methods aim to detect functional loss by using a range of chromatic, contrast, static and dynamic stimuli alone or in combination.

2.3.3. Most common types of AP

1. Short-Wave Automated Perimetry (SWAP)

SWAP is a visual field test procedure that is designed to isolate and measure the visual pathway mechanisms that are maximally sensitive to short wavelength (blue) light. This is accomplished by superimposing a large (Goldmann Size V) short wavelength (blue) target on a bright (100 candelas per meter squared) yellow background. The bright yellow background decreases the sensitivity of the middle (green) and long (red) wavelength mechanisms. Several studies have demonstrated that SWAP is able to detect glaucomatous and neuro-ophthalmologic visual field loss in eyes with standard white-on-white automated perimetry (SAP) within normal limits, demonstrates deficits that are larger than for SAP, and identifies progression earlier than SAP.[34-40] Optimal test procedures have also been determined.[41] However, other studies from independent laboratories have reported that SWAP is not able to detect glaucomatous visual field loss or progression any better than SAP.[42-44]

2. Frequency Doubling Technology (FDT) & Humphrey Matrix FDT Perimetry

The presentation of a low spatial frequency sinusoidal grating (less than two cycles per degree of visual angle) at a high rate of counterphase alternation (flicker) of greater than 15 Hertz (cycles per second) produces the appearance of approximately twice as many light and dark bars than are physically present. This has resulted in the phenomenon being referred to as the frequency doubling effect. A device for evaluation of visual field loss produced by glaucoma and other ocular and neurologic diseases was developed and referred to as the frequency doubling technology (FDT) perimeter. It presents 10 degree by 10 degree targets at 19 locations throughout the central 30 degree (radius) visual field that had a spatial frequency of 0.25 cycles per degree and flickered at 25 Hertz. The contrast of the targets is altered to determine the minimum contrast needed to detect the FDT target from a uniform background. A second generation device, known as the Humphrey Matrix, was subsequently developed that reduced the size of the targets (5 degrees by 5 degrees) to provide additional features as well as the ability to test up to 68 locations to allow tests to be performed with the 30-2, 24-2, 10-2 and macula stimulus configurations. To accomplish this, the target's spatial frequency was increased to 0.5 cycles per degree and the temporal frequency was reduced to 18 Hertz. Both devices have normative databases and statistical analysis packages, and have been reported to be useful in detecting and following visual field loss from glaucoma and other ocular and neurological diseases.[3,45-51] FDT perimetry has similar diagnostic precision as SAP for the identification of glaucoma.[44]

3. Flicker Perimetry

Flicker perimetry consists of presentation of a target the luminance of which is alternated from light to dark for a particular temporal frequency. Currently, there are four different forms of flicker perimetry: (1) determination of the highest rate of flicker that can be detected for a high contrast target (Critical flicker frequency or CFF); (2) evaluation of the minimum amount of contrast needed to detect flicker for a specified temporal frequency (temporal modulation perimetry); (3) measurement of the minimum luminance of a background pedestal to detect a flickering target superimposed on the background pedestal (luminance pedestal flicker); and (4) determination of the minimum amount of contrast of a group of flickering dots 180 degrees out of phase with a larger group of dots (flicker-defined form, as performed on the Heidelberg Edge Perimeter [HEP]).[52-54] Each of the flicker procedures has its particular advantages and disadvantages, but all have been shown to be effective in early detection of visual field loss.[55-57] Luminance pedestal flicker can produce confusion for elderly patients with visual impairment who confuse onset of a steady target versus with perceived flicker, thereby producing response errors. A comparison of CFF perimetry and temporal modulation perimetry was performed in a group of glaucoma patients, and it was found that temporal modulation perimetry has modestly better performance (greater area under the Receiver Operating Curve for distinguishing healthy normal controls from glaucoma patients) than CFF perimetry.[52] One advantage of flicker perimetry is that it is not affected by refractive error or optical aberrations as much as other forms of perimetric testing.[57]

4. Flicker-Defined Form Perimetry (Heidelberg Edge Perimetry, HEP)

The method uses a contrast, flicker-defined form stimulus that produces an illusionary edge perceived at the border of two random dot areas that modulate in counter-phase at a high temporal frequency of 15 Hz, and an adaptive staircase thresholding algorithm (ASTA) strategy.[54,58-60]

HEP dynamic range is lower than SAP.[61] Hence this technique is limited to early glaucoma diagnosis. Learning and fatigue effects have been reported in healthy subjects.[63]

Studies performed with ocular hypertensives, glaucoma suspects and early glaucoma patients have reported that HEP may identify visual field loss in subjects with normal SAP.[61-64] However, such study design does not allow for the detection of abnormal SAP in subjects with normal HEP. In one report including ocular hypertensives and glaucoma patients diagnosed only by optic disc appearance, and healthy subjects required to have normal SAP, HEP results were classified as abnormal in more glaucoma patients than SAP. Findings support a higher sensitivity of HEP to detect functional damage than SAP when concurrently abnormal spectral domain optical coherence tomography (SDOCT) retinal nerve fiber layer thickness (RNFLT) measurements are found, although specificity was not reported.[61] In another study, HEP had significant correlations with structural parameters measured with Heidelberg retinal tomography (HRT) in glaucomatous and healthy eyes.[65]

HEP sensitivity appears to be comparable to FDT and RNFLT measured with SDOCT in early glaucoma at a fixed specificity level, according to one study.[66]

5. Kinetic Perimetry

Kinetic perimetry uses test targets that are fixed in size and luminance. They are moved from non-seeing areas into seeing portions of the visual field, and the limits of the visual field are mapped using different size and luminance target combinations. The Goldmann perimeter is a common device for kinetic perimetry (note that the original Haag-Streit Goldmann perimeter is no longer being manufactured, but compatible devices are available) and some automated perimeters have a computer-assisted semi-automated kinetic program.

The advantages of kinetic perimetry include that (1) the full extent of the visual field can be tested with the same strategy in a short time; (2) it is useful for mapping the shape and pattern of visual field defects; (3) it is useful for advanced stages of diseases and subjects with poor acuity;[67-69] (4) it is acceptable for children,[70-73] elderly and unreliable subjects; (5) it may identify peripheral defects in 4-10% of glaucoma patients with a normal central field;[74-78] (6) it is useful for assessment of the quality of vision required for driving.[79]

The disadvantages of manual kinetic perimetry include that (1) it requires a highly-trained perimetrist; (2) reproducibility is poor among examiners and institutions;[80] and (3) it does not provide numerical data for comparison.

Recently, computer-assisted semi-automated kinetic perimetry has become available for Octopus perimeters and several other automated perimeters. Compatibility with the Goldmann perimeter[81,82] and basic studies for kinetic approaches, such as learning and fatigue effects, and the effects of stimulus velocity and target size and of pupil size, stray light and defocus, have been reported using semi-automated kinetic methods.[83-93] In some automated perimeters, the peripheral visual field limits that can be tested are not compatible with the original Goldmann perimeter.

Additional advantages of semi-automated kinetic perimetry are (1) target speed is exactly controlled by the perimeter; (2) isopter area is automatically calculated and quantitative analysis is available; (3) age-matched normal values are provided; (4) the patient's reaction time is measured to adjust the responses to obtain more accurate and reproducible results;[94-96] and (5) all kinetic procedures can be recorded and used for the next examination.

However, there are still limitations of semi-automated kinetic perimetry. The results are still dependent on the examiners' skill. Several computer-based simulation studies and new, fully automated kinetic algorithms have been reported.[81,97,98] Furthermore, the kinetic approach is a time consuming strategy especially in the central 30-degree visual field if the detailed shape of a scotoma is needed. It was reported that a combination of central static perimetry and peripheral kinetic perimetry appears to be one of the practical approaches to this issue.[99,100]

6. Motion Perimetry

The ability to detect motion is a prominent attribute of visual function, especially in the periphery. There are generally two forms of motion perimetry testing that have been introduced: (1) determination of the minimum displacement of a single target needed to detection motion (displacement threshold perimetry); and (2) assessment of the motion or direction of a subset of dots within a larger group of stationary or randomly moving dots (motion coherence thresholds).[101-107] Motion perimetry is a robust visual function that is relatively unaffected by refractive error, contrast, background luminance and many other factors, which makes it particularly suitable for clinical testing.[108] Motion perimetry is an effective procedure for glaucoma detection,[109,110] and is a preferred procedure by most patients.

7. Pulsar Perimetry

This method combines contrast and spatial resolution stimuli, either moving or pulsed. The standard characteristics used in glaucoma diagnosis include white light, temporal modulation at 30 Hz in phase and counter-phase, namely T30W, and a tendency oriented perimetry (TOP) strategy.[111] The unit of measurement is the 'src', derived from its capacity to measure spatial resolution (sr) and contrast (c).

Pulsar peripheral and central dynamic ranges have been reported as narrower and comparable to SAP, respectively.[114,115] Fluctuations are lower than SAP.[112] Learning effects appear to be not significant in patients with previous SAP experience.[113,114]

Pulsar perimetry has been focused mainly on the detection of early glaucomatous functional loss. Studies performed with Pulsar in ocular hypertensives, glaucoma suspects and early glaucoma patients have suggested this method can be useful to detect early functional loss.[115-118]

Pulsar sensitivity has been reported to be better than FDT in early glaucoma in one study[119] and comparable to detect functional loss at a fixed specificity level than FDT and rarebit perimetry in another study.[120]

8. Rarebit Perimetry

Rarebit perimetry is a test procedure that presents small bright (supra-threshold) targets on a dark background that are displayed on a calibrated computer monitor. The observer's task is to determine whether there were zero, one or two dots that were presented simultaneously on the display screen and to click a mouse button zero, one or two times to indicate the number of targets seen. A variety of different patterns is available for evaluation of the central 30-degree radius visual field or the macular region. By using a combination of various dot configurations, Rarebit perimetry attempts to provide fine detail mapping of visual field detection of the targets by calculating the hit rate for each location tested. It has been reported to be useful in identifying visual field loss in glaucoma and other retinal and optic nerve diseases, it can be implemented on any PC, and it may be useful in identifying heterogeneous or 'patchy' visual field loss.[121-125]

9. Size Threshold Perimetry

The use of the Goldmann perimeter for performing kinetic perimetry was instrumental in establishing target size as an important variable in visual field testing. However, with the advent of SAP, the use of a fixed target size (typically a Goldmann Size III, but sometimes a size V for cases of advanced visual field loss) became standard. The Heidelberg Edge Perimeter (HEP) varies the target size according to the visual field eccentricity of the target (large targets for more peripheral locations),[52] and recent studies have introduced varying target size as a means of altering target visibility.[126] Recent reports indicate that this procedure is as effective as conventional SAP testing, and is often preferred by patients as a diagnostic test procedure.[126]

All perimetry tests exhibit marked between-subject and test-retest variability; studies evaluating alternative perimetry are more informative if the signal-to-noise ratio of the tests relative to SAP is reported.[126]

2.4. Progression analysis for diagnosis

Andrew McNaught, Stuart Gardiner, David Garway-Heath

2.4.1. Research needs

Further research would be valuable to identify the optimal statistical analysis of both structure and function in early glaucoma, probably using novel statistical approaches, which exploit the valuable information available from both.

2.4.2. Use of SAP to detect functional glaucoma damage

Detection of the earliest functional glaucoma damage in patients at risk of developing glaucoma is challenging, even in patients with already clear evidence of structural glaucoma damage. The current standard for the detection of functional damage is still standard automated perimetry (SAP). The HFA is now a prevalent device in ophthalmology units: 99% of UK eye departments use some form of automated perimetry, 78% having the HFA.[127] In a survey of UK community optometrists,[128] the perimeter most frequently used was either one of the Henson range of instruments (39%) or the Humphrey Field Analyser (22%). The HFA is used by both general ophthalmologists, and has been extensively used in research trials such as AGIS, CIGTS, EMGT, OHTS, as well as the more recently completed UKGTS trial.[129] There has been extensive research confirming the value of SAP, mainly using the HFA, Octopus, or Henson perimeters, in the detection, and monitoring, of glaucomatous visual function progression: using both ‘event’ and ‘trend’ analysis in the analysis of global indices, as well as point-wise techniques.[130]

2.4.3. Alternatives to SAP to detect early evidence of deterioration in visual function

A. Short-wavelength perimetry (SWAP)

This perimetry technique features a blue stimulus on yellow background. The theoretical advantage underpinning this mode of visual function testing is the relatively less dense matrix of blue cones serving the central visual field: this ‘reduced redundancy’ may lead to earlier glaucomatous losses being detectable using shorter wavelength stimuli. Research work by several groups has highlighted higher long-term fluctuation than SAP, and probably more of a marked confounding effect of cataract. The higher long-term fluctuation characteristic of SWAP theoretically reduces the appeal of SWAP in the detection of VF progression. Reports have been published which suggest that SWAP is able to detect glaucomatous progression prior to SAP. More recent work by Van de Schoot *et al.*[131] has not supported this: in a study of 416 ocular hypertensive subjects, 24 eyes of 21 subjects showed conversion using SAP. Of these eyes, 22 did not show earlier conversion in SWAP than with SAP. SAP even demonstrated earlier conversion than SWAP in 15 cases. In only two eyes did SWAP show earlier conversion by up to 18 months. SAP appears to be at least as sensitive to functional conversion to glaucoma as SWAP in a large majority of eyes. SWAP is now considered less valuable for the detection, and monitoring, of glaucomatous progression.

B. Frequency-doubling technology (FDT) perimetry

This rapid visual function test was designed to exploit the frequency doubling illusion. Early work has demonstrated a sensitivity of 85%, and a specificity of 90% for the detection of 'early glaucoma' using the HFA as 'gold-standard'.[132] There has been limited work to ascertain if FDT is suitable for detecting progression. A recent study by Xin *et al.*[133] enrolled 33 glaucoma patients (55 eyes). The following tests were performed at two baseline and follow-up exams: FDT, 24-2 HVF, multi-focal visual evoked potentials, optical coherence tomography and stereo-photographs. There was 21.1 (± 1.8 months) follow-up. For HVF there were significant changes in MD in eight (14.5%) eyes. For FDT, there were significant changes in MD in 13 (23.6%) eyes. Only five eyes showed changes in MD for both HVF and FDT. Each test showed progression in some eyes, but agreement among tests on which eyes showed progression was poor. In a further study by Fan *et al.*,[134] in eyes with SAP within normal limits, of patients with OAG, FDT detected visual field loss in almost two of every three of these eyes and also predicted to some extent future visual field loss on SAP. However, a study has not yet been performed looking at the predictive value of SAP in eyes with normal FDT. A further study by Haymes *et al.*[135] compared the prevalence of functional progression using SAP compared with FDT (C-20/N-30 programs) in 65 patients who were followed for a median of 3.5 years (median number of examinations, 9). 32 (49%) patients were found to have progressing visual fields with FDT, and 32 (49%) patients with SAP. Only 16 (25%) patients showed progression with both methods. There is only limited evidence, to date, guiding the use of FDT perimeter in the early detection of glaucomatous progression. Meira-Freitas *et al.*[51] showed that the rate of change of FDT PSD was predictive of development of a repeatable SAP defect among eyes that did not have such a defect at baseline, even after accounting for the rate of SAP PSD change. They also suggested that FDT PSD may have started to change sooner than SAP PSD among eyes that subsequently progressed. However, the FDT Matrix has a more limited number of possible sensitivity values (15 in total) than SAP, with large gaps between some of the possibilities. So far, there is no convincing data suggesting a difference in the ability of the SAP and FDT perimeters to measure progression.

C. Motion sensitivity

Motion sensitivity measures the sensitivity of the patient to a moving stimulus within the central visual field. Tests of motion, lacking any resolution component, constitute a 'hyper-acuity' test,[136] and are more robust to the effects of cataract and blur.[108] An early version of the test, which tested a single visual field location, did show some potential value in the early detection of functional motion defects, which preceded SAP defects with a sensitivity of 75%, and a specificity of 84%.[103] More recent work has described further development of a multi-location motion sensitivity test,[137] but there is no published work, as yet, describing use in the monitoring of glaucoma progression.

There is currently insufficient evidence to recommend the use of motion sensitivity in detecting early visual field progression.

2.4.4. Evidence to support use of progression analysis to detect function loss prior to standard definitions of SAP functional damage

There is limited evidence exploring the potential for use of progression analysis of series of SAP results in eyes considered at risk of developing functional loss, but with no clear evidence of existing visual field loss, using generally accepted visual field staging systems. It seems reasonable to suggest that if an eye initially had sensitivities towards the upper end of the (quite wide) normal range, then progression may be detectable before the sensitivity becomes outside normal limits by any metric; however empirical evidence to support this proposition is lacking. *Scientific evidence supporting the common clinical practice of simply observing the patient who is suspected of having glaucoma, (perhaps with risk factors, for example, relatively high IOP, and a family history), but with equivocal structural measurements, over time, to see if any evidence of progressive (functional) glaucomatous damage can be established, would be useful to support this practice in those many cases of diagnostic uncertainty.*

Two principal patient groups have been studied, which might reasonably be expected to be at enhanced risk of visual field loss appearing, even if the initial functional measurements fall within normal limits. The groups comprise *ocular hypertensive* patients, and also patients with normal tension glaucoma (NTG) considered at particular risk of developing visual field damage, *i.e., the initially normal fellow eyes of eyes with clear evidence of NTG in the fellow eye.*

2.4.4.1. Ocular hypertensive patients (OHT)

A key study by Demirel *et al.*[138] examining data from the Ocular Hypertension Treatment Study (OHTS), considered the rate of decay in HFA mean deviation (MD) across the participants in the OHTS study, broken down into groups defined by the eventual clinical outcome, *i.e.*, whether the eye developed a trial endpoint, whether that endpoint was defined by visual field defect development with or without a structural endpoint, and whether that patient was in the intervention or non-intervention group. The mean and median rate of MD decay in the subgroups is summarized in Table 1 (reproduced from the original report): interestingly, but perhaps not surprisingly, the rate of MD decay was faster in the subgroup that eventually developed a visual field conversion endpoint, and more rapid yet in the subgroup that developed both visual field and structural endpoints. Another interesting finding was that in those eyes that developed any study endpoint (visual field or structure) that signaled conversion to glaucoma, there was no significant difference in the MD decay rate between those that were treated and those who were in the non-intervention group.

Quoting from the authors: '*Perhaps, the most striking finding from this study was that the mean MDR in eyes with ocular hypertension, including those that converted to POAG, was slow (−0.08 dB/y). At this rate it would take approximately three decades for a visual field to progress from the normal mean (MD = 0 dB) to the 5th percentile of a healthy reference group (MD ≈ −2.2 dB).*' This is an important observation, in that, if one was to use rate of MD decay in OHT patients as a key indicator of impending development of a visual field defect which would satisfy most definitions of damage, the fact that the rate of loss is quite slow (when compared with the rate of loss found in other studies in glaucoma, *e.g.*, EMGT), might suggest that regression analysis of MD might not be of great clinical utility as an 'early warning sign' in OHT. However, MDR was significantly worse in those eyes that reached an endpoint (mean -0.26 dB/yr) than in those

Table 2. Rates of change of Mean deviation (MDR) in dB/yr for different categories of eyes.

OHTS Classification	N (eyes)	Rate of MD decay (dB/year) mean	95% CL about mean	Mean	2.5%	97%
All eyes	2609	-0.08	-0.08 – -0.07	-0.5	-0.52	0.19
No POAG endpoint	2250	-0.05	-0.05 – -0.04	-0.04	-0.35	0.20
All POAG (optic disc and/ or VF change	359	-0.26	-0.30 – -0.22	-0.17	-1.31	0.12
POAG due to VF change only	74	-0.29	-0.36 – -0.22	-0.22	-1.21	0.07
POAG due to optic disc change only	158	-.012	-0.15 – -0.09	-0.09	-0.60	0.13
POAG due to either VF OR optic disc change	232	-0.17	-0.20 – -0.14	-0.12	0.90	0.13
POAG due to both VF AND optic disc change	127	-0.42	-0.50 – -0.34	-0.27	-1.98	0.05
Randomized to observation in OHTS phase 1	1302	-0.08	-0.10 – -0.07	-0.05	-0.55	0.19
Randomized to treatment in OHTS phase 1	1307	-0.07	-0.08 – -0.06	-0.05	-0.46	0.19

CI = Confidence interval; POAG = Primary open-angle glaucoma; VF = Visual field.

that did not (mean -0.05 dB/yr), suggesting that, while on average MD does not change quickly, it may be useful for early identification of rapid progression. In conclusion, as the authors argue convincingly in the manuscript, since the earliest visual field defects are often, but not always, focal defects, the use of MD may not be the most efficient use of the available visual field data: MD is especially good at detecting a general fall in field sensitivity, but is less good at detecting focal losses, which, by definition, will have little impact on the global index that is MD.

Addressing this point, a similar study, also using data from OHTS, by Artes *et al.*[139] compared change probability analysis of MD decay versus similar analysis of pattern standard deviation (PSD) decay in visual field data from 3088 eyes of 1570 subjects who were enrolled in the OHTS. The authors also looked at cross-sectional criteria for field progression, including the Glaucoma Hemifield Test (GHT). The authors found that both cross-sectional and longitudinal analyses of PSD were more conservative than analyses of MD, with a three- to five-fold lower incidence of progression, whether measured using a cross-sectional, or trend technique. Further work addressing early losses appearing in glaucoma suspects needs to be sensitive to both an overall decline in field sensitivity, as well as focal field defects.

2.4.4.2. Initially functionally normal fellow eyes in NTG patients

There has been a small number of reports describing the natural history of functional progression in the initially functionally normal fellow eyes of patients with confirmed NTG in the other eye. One of the earliest reports was by Baez *et al.*,[140] who described the use of motion sensitivity testing to attempt to detect focal functional loss prior to SAP abnormality. The motion sensitivity test showed modest power to predict the subsequent development of a focal SAP defect in initially functionally normal fellow eyes of NTG patients. An interesting observation was the likelihood of visual field defect development in these initially normal NTG fellow eyes: '*In 22 of the 51 eyes (43%) with normal visual fields at presentation, field deterioration occurred at one or more Humphrey locations within a mean of 1.7 (SD 1.6) years.*'

A much lower rate of visual field defect development was reported by Cho *et al.*[141] in a similar study of initially normal NTG fellow eyes, namely 6%: 'Among six patients (12%) who had developed either RNFL defect or NRR notching, only three patients (6%) developed VF loss in 1.81, 3.09, and 9.27 years.'

Finally, a study by Membrey *et al.*[142] demonstrated that 36.4% of initially functionally normal NTG fellow eyes developed visual field progression using point-wise linear regression analysis.

2.4.5. Discussion

There is currently only a small evidence base to inform the usefulness of progression analysis of SAP measurements to attempt to anticipate the development of a visual field defect in an eye with an initially normal SAP result. SAP analysis techniques, which could be used to deliver this potentially clinically useful tool, would have to be sensitive to the development of both generalized and focal sensitivity loss. Simply undertaking regression analysis of MD may not capture the earliest progression of focal visual field loss. However, Artes *et al.*[139] showed that if focal field loss alone is sought, the sensitivity for detecting early functional loss is much lower, as some subjects converting from OHT to glaucoma will have general reduction in visual field sensitivity as the sole functional indicator of conversion. The evidence from NTG fellow eyes is less conclusive, but the evidence that is available suggests, in any case, that the risk of visual field defect appearance is anything between 43%,[140] over approximately two years follow-up) and 6%,[141] over nine years), though this wide range no doubt also reflects differences in the definition of visual field loss between studies.

The clinical need to reliably anticipate the development of the patients first visual field defect is arguable: if the visual field results are equivocal, the clinician always has complementary evidence from the structural measurements, *i.e.*, the presence or absence of ONH or RNFL damage. However, a study by Strouthidis *et al.*[143] in a different study of OHT subjects, examining both functional and structural progression (using neuro-retinal rim are) showed, quoting from the authors: '*A relatively high frequency of detected disease progression was observed with either method, with progression by VF occurring at least as frequently as progression by RA. Poor agreement between RA and VF progression was observed regardless of the specificity of the progression criteria. The results indicate that, in patients with ocular hypertension, monitoring of both VF and optic disc is necessary, as agreement between optic disc and VF progression is the exception rather than the rule*'.

2.4.6. Conclusion

In clinical practice, considering the patient with OHT, with, by definition, normal visual fields, or the NTG patient with obvious glaucoma damage in the fellow eye, the presence of clinically certain structural damage in the eye with an apparently normal visual field might usually suggest the need for treatment. Detection of functional progression should be sufficient evidence to diagnose glaucoma, even if the visual field remains within normal limits (especially if the field was initially towards the high end of the normal range); but it is not a necessary criterion, since methods to detect progression are not yet sufficiently sensitive and accurate. Nonetheless, further research into developing better methods to fully utilize the rich data available in a long series of even apparently normal (if analyzed in isolation) SAP results, in concert with the structural measures, from a patient with risk factors for eventual functional damage would seem worthwhile.

2.5. Electrophysiology

Donald Hood, Carlos Gustavo De Moraes, Brad Fortune

2.5.1. Research Needs

1. Studies are needed to elucidate the source and mechanisms of reversible aspects of functional loss measured by PERG and PhNR testing.
2. Studies are needed to determine the extent to which PERG and PhNR signals depend on intact glial cell function in the retina and optic nerve head (*i.e.*, can PERG and PhNR abnormalities be considered strictly a reflection of retinal ganglion cell function or are they also influenced independently by change in glial cell physiology?).
3. Further studies are needed to determine more precisely the positive (and negative) predictive value of PERG and PhNR testing for subsequent glaucoma progression and whether there is a value added to the current standard combinations of visual field testing and OCT imaging.

2.5.2. Pattern Electroretinogram (PERG)

The pattern electroretinogram (PERG) is the most well-established ERG technique for studying glaucoma (for reviews of PERG historical background and utility for glaucoma diagnosis see references 144-149).

The results of two recently published PERG studies serve well to characterize the potential utility of the PERG for glaucoma management. The first of these studies, by Banitt and colleagues,[150] evaluated longitudinal rates of change for peripapillary retinal nerve fiber layer (RNFL) thickness and PERG amplitude in glaucoma suspects. They found that the glaucoma suspect eyes with the smallest baseline PERG amplitude (≤ 50% of its age-adjusted normative value) had the fastest rate of RNFL thickness decline over the subsequent five years.[150] Banitt *et al.* concluded that a glaucoma suspect with a severely reduced PERG indicates a need for "*closer monitoring or treatment as he or she will have a higher rate of RNFL thinning.*"

The second recently published noteworthy study was by Bode *et al.* who found that the PERG "detected glaucoma patients 4 years before visual field changes occurred, with a sensitivity/specificity of 75%/76%."[151] Another interesting finding from their study was that the predictive capacity of PERG for eventual conversion from normal to glaucomatous visual field damage "*was roughly constant from conversion to 4 years before conversion, fitting with the view that PERG changes occur early and then saturate, thus rendering the PERG a poor biomarker for monitoring advanced disease.*" Although the outcome measure in the Bode *et al.* study was visual field conversion, their result has a similar implication to the observation by Banitt *et al.*[150] In particular, RNFL thickness does not exhibit loss until PERG amplitude is severely reduced. The results of both studies imply that PERG amplitude cannot decline much further beyond initial detectable loss and would thus not be useful for monitoring moderate-to-advanced glaucoma.

The evidence from this pair of studies suggest that the PERG may be most beneficial as an adjunct in the diagnosis and management of glaucoma suspects (with normal or near normal visual fields and/or RNFL thickness) by helping to stratify risk: for those suspect eyes with a severely reduced PERG (and no other evidence of outer retinal dysfunction), it may be prudent to increase frequency of follow-up and/or initiate therapy.

One important caveat is that the PERG, like any test of RGC function, depends on a cascade of intact outer retinal signals, so without a focal macular ERG or multifocal ERG to evaluate specifically the macular cone and cone bipolar responses, the PERG alone is not a specific assay of RGC function; the PERG will yield abnormal findings in patients with middle and outer retinal damage. This is important as most glaucoma patients are older and may exhibit concomitant age-related decline of outer retinal function too. In addition, as the PERG is a small signal, it is prone to interference from environmental noise and blinking artifact. Although it is independent of patient motor and cognitive skills (unlike perimetry), it still requires careful control of fixation, refraction, and stimulus distance and is best performed under the supervision of an electrophysiologist that has expertise with PERG recordings. Yet, even under ideal recording conditions, there can be substantial inter-individual variability of PERG amplitude and overlap between healthy and glaucomatous eyes.[151,152] Thus the PERG is likely to offer high positive predictive value, but not necessarily high negative predictive value.

2.5.3. Photopic Negative Response (PhNR)

The PhNR is a slow negative component that manifests after the b-wave of the cone driven full-field ERG, as first characterized by Viswanathan *et al.*[153,154] Like the PERG, the PhNR is dependent on intact RGC responses, which in turn also depend on intact feed-forward responses of cone photoreceptor and cone bipolar neurons.[153,154] Since the PhNR is elicited by a uniform full-field stimulus, in contrast to the PERG, it is not as critically dependent on accurate refraction, clear optics or exquisite fixation control, which is potentially advantageous for clinical testing. Another distinct advantage over the PERG is that the PhNR enables simultaneous assessment of distal retinal function (cone photoreceptor and cone bipolar cell responses) from the same recording. However, the reliability and diagnostic efficacy of the PhNR are likely improved by recording with dilated pupils, unlike the PERG, which is a disadvantage for clinical testing. Because the PhNR is also a newer technique than PERG, there is even less consensus on the best protocol to use for glaucoma in terms of stimulus characteristics (intensity and chromaticity) and signal analysis (amplitude measurement details). An excellent review of PhNR clinical applications was published by Machida in 2012.[155]

Since the review by Machida in 2012, several other PhNR studies relevant to glaucoma have been published. For example, Niyadurupola and collegues[156] demonstrated improvement in the PhNR amplitude within one to two months of IOP lowering by standard clinical therapy for glaucoma. In contrast, eyes that did not achieve significant IOP reduction (< 25% reduction) did not have any change in PhNR amplitude over the same period.

More recently, Machida and colleagues[157] used a focal stimulation technique to evaluate regional variation within the macula of the relationship between A-wave, B-wave and PhNR amplitudes and the thickness of the ganglion cell complex measured by spectral domain optical coherence tomography (SD-OCT) in glaucoma. They found that the PhNR was more prominent in the central macular ERG responses (15 degrees) as compared with responses elicited by annular stimuli around the macula (15-30 degrees). Further, Machida *et al.*[157] found that PhNR amplitudes were well correlated with the thickness of the ganglion cell complex within the central macula, but only weakly correlated outside of the central macula. However, one aspect of their data that the investigators did not mention is the fact that there was much more overlap between open-angle glaucoma and healthy eyes for PhNR amplitude (and PhNR/b-wave amplitude ratio) than there was for the ganglion cell complex measured by SD-OCT. This means that the diagnostic utility of the PhNR is substantially lower than OCT measurements of ganglion cell complex thickness (a fast and completely non-invasive test). In fact, in their paper, there were very few examples of glaucoma eyes with a normal ganglion cell complex thickness but abnormal focal PhNR amplitude.

In general, concerning the value of the ERG to the clinician faced with glaucoma diagnosis and management, we believe there is a very limited role.

This role includes objective assessment of RGC function, limited to the central macula in early stages of glaucoma (including suspects). In such cases, with or without subjective complaints of vision impairment, a markedly reduced PERG or PhNR (preferably focal or multifocal for the central 15 degrees) is indicative of RGC dysfunction and warrants careful follow-up and potentially therapeutic intervention, especially when accompanied by evidence of structural loss (such as thinning of the macular inner retinal layers, reduction of peripapillary RNFL thickness, progressive optic disc changes and/or splinter hemorrhages). In this regard, the PERG and PhNR may serve to help stratify risk for glaucoma progression, no doubt an important consideration. The converging evidence that PERG and PhNR measurements may also reveal some reversible aspect of glaucomatous dysfunction has important implications; future studies will hopefully uncover the source and mechanism of these effects.

2.5.4. Multifocal Visual Evoked Potential (mfVEP)

The mfVEP is far superior to any form of ERG for objective topographic assessment of vision function in glaucoma.[158-163] However, it should be noted that, in general, the diagnostic accuracy of mfVEP is about the same as psychophysical perimetry.[158-163] Even though false-positive results are inherent of any diagnostic technique, previous reports of the mfVEP technique have shown approximately a 3% rate,[164] as well as fairly good sensitivity and specificity compared with other technologies.

Given its objective nature, the mfVEP technique could be valuable in categorizing subjects with unreliable, unconfirmed or excessively variable SAP field defects. Fortune *et al.*[161] found that the classification by mfVEP and SAP results agreed in 75–81% of early glaucomatous eyes. A more detailed comparison reveals that the mfVEP will often detect scotomata that are missed by 24-2 perimetry, but seen using a 10-2 test pattern, since the mfVEP stimulus typically has a high density of test locations within the central 10 degrees. One study found that, in eyes with normal-tension glaucoma, the mfVEP confirmed 92% of the central scotomata seen on SAP. Moreover, the mfVEP showed central abnormalities in 44% of the eyes with apparently preserved central function on SAP.[162] On one hand, some of these abnormalities could be false-positive results due to poor fixation or low signal-to-noise during mfVEP testing. On the other hand, eyes with normal-tension glaucoma tend to present with central defects more often than eyes with high-tension glaucoma,[165] so it is possible that the mfVEP has a better sensitivity to detect central abnormalities. In contrast, the mfVEP may miss defects in the upper hemifield that manifest as arcuate defects by 24-2 perimetry, largely because of the anatomical configuration of primary visual cortex relative to the position of the surface electrodes used for recording.

The objective nature of the technique offers an advantage over psychophysical tests of visual function. In glaucoma suspects or ocular hypertensives with unreliable or inconclusive SAP results, a normal mfVEP result can help rule out functional damage and thus have a strong effect on clinical decisions. Conversely, an abnormal mfVEP result could be considered a true finding, particularly when corroborated by topographically matched optic nerve findings (*i.e.*, optic disc photography or OCT).

2.6. Staging algorithms

Paolo Brusini, Remo Susanna Jr, David Crabb, Ryo Asaoka

The classification of glaucomatous VF defect severity is an important issue for several reasons, which include: having consistent criteria when perimetry is used to define glaucoma damage severity, providing a reference for deciding treatment intensity on the basis of disease severity, describing VF results in a short and simple format, and providing a common language in clinical and research settings. Several classification methods have been proposed in the past, using both standard automated perimetry (SAP) and some non-conventional perimetric techniques such as Frequency Doubling Technology. A review on this topic has been published some years ago in Survey Ophthalmology.[166] In this review, all the methods available at that time are reported and critically discussed.

Among the methods discussed, only four are currently widely used to stage the visual field damage severity:

1. The Hodapp-Anderson-Parrish and (H-A-P) classification,[167] based on two criteria: (a) the overall extent of damage, which is calculated from both the MD value and the number of defective points in the Humphrey Statpac-2 pattern deviation probability map of the 30-2 full threshold test; and (b) the defect proximity to the fixation point. The defect extent is summarized in three classes (early, moderate, and advanced) (Table 3).

Table 3. The Hodapp-Anderson-Parrish classification.

EARLY DEFECT:
• MD < -6 dB • < 25% p < 5% points and < 10 p < 1% points (pattern deviation) • no point < 15 dB within the central 5°
MODERATE DEFECT:
• MD < -12 dB • < 50% p < 5% points and < 20 p < 1% points • no 0 dB point within the central 5° • only a hemifield with one point < 15 dB within the central 5°
ADVANCED DEFECT:
• MD > -12 dB • > 50% p < 5% points or > 20 p < 1% points • some 0 dB points within the central 5° • some < 15 dB points in both hemifields within the central 5°

2. The Advanced Glaucoma Intervention Study (AGIS) visual field defect score,[168] based on both the number and depth of adjacent depressed test locations in various sub-divisions of the visual field (Fig. 4). The AGIS score is calculated looking at the total deviation plot of the Statpac 2 single field analysis (24-2 threshold test). Visual field scores, ranging between 0 and 20, are divided in five stages. The Collaborative Initial Glaucoma Treatment Trial (CIGTS) proposed in 1999 a similar classification method.[169]

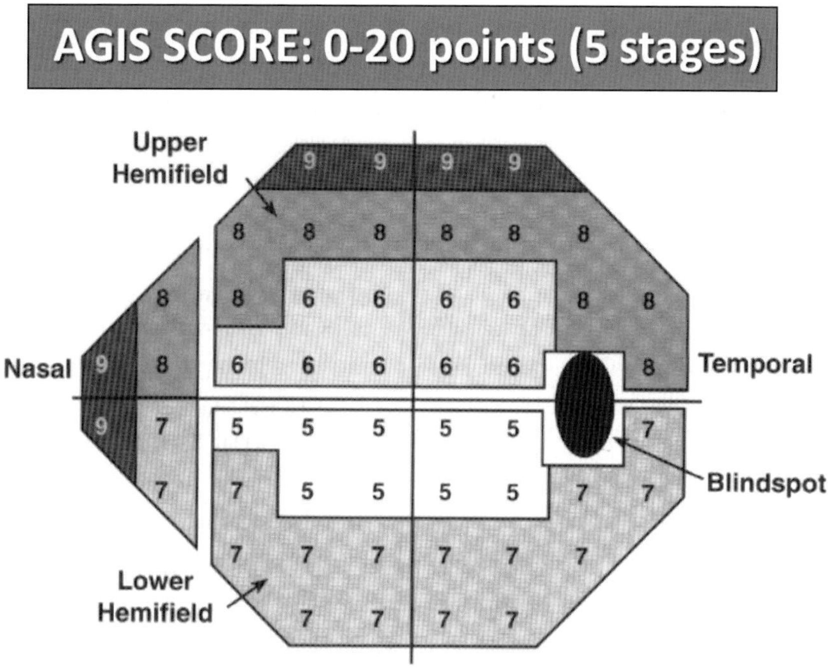

Fig. 4. Advanced Glaucoma Intervention Study scoring template.

3. The Bascom-Palmer Visual Field Staging System, proposed by Mills *et al.* in 2006,[170] which takes into consideration the MD and CPSD/PSD values, the number of disturbed points in the pattern probability map, the presence or not of a very depressed point near fixation, and the GHT result (for stage 1) (Table 4). This method, which appears to be an enhanced version of the H-A-P classification, is detailed, but is too time-consuming to be used in a clinical setting.

4. The Glaucoma Staging System (GSS) version 1 and 2, introduced by Brusini in 1996 and 2006,[171,172] respectively, which uses the MD and the CPSD/CLV (or CLV/LV) values on a Cartesian coordinate diagram (Fig. 5). This graph allows the user to simultaneously know the disease severity (classified in six stages), and the

Table 4: The Bascom-Palmer Visual Field Staging System.

Stage
Stage 0: No or minimal defect/ocular hypertension Does not meet any criteria for stage 1.
Stage 1: Early defect MD ≥ -6.00 dB and at least one of the following: A. On pattern deviation plot, there exists a cluster of 3 or more points in an expected location of the visual field depressed below the 5% level, at least 1 of which is depressed below the 1% level B. Corrected pattern standard deviation/pattern standard deviation significant P < 0.05 C. Glaucoma hemifield test "Outside Normal Limits"
Stage 2: Moderate defect MD of -6.01 to -12.00 dB and at least one of the following: A. On pattern deviation plot, greater than or equal to 25% but fewer than 50% of points depressed below the 5% level, and greater than or equal to 15% but fewer than 25% of points depressed below the 1% B. At least 1 point within central 5° with sensitivity of <15 dB but, no point within central 5° with sensitivity of < 0 dB C. Only 1 hemifield containing a point with sensitivity < 15 dB within 5° of fixation
Stage 3: Advanced defect MD of -12.01 dB to -20.00 dB and at least one of the following: A. On pattern deviation plot, greater than or equal to 50% but fewer than 75% of points depressed below the 5% level and greater than or equal to 25% but fewer than 50% of points depressed below 1% level B. Any point within central 5° with sensitivity of < 0 dB C. Both hemifields containing a point(s) with sensitivity < 15 dB within 5° of fixation
Stage 4: Severe defect MD of -20.00 dB and at least one of the following: A. On pattern deviation plot, greater than or equal to 75% of points depressed below the 5% level and greater than or equal to 50% of points depressed below 1% level B. At least 50% of points within central 5° with sensitivity of < 0 dB C. Both hemifields containing greater than 50% of points with sensitivity < 15 dB within 5 degrees of fixation
Stage 5: End-stage disease Unable to perform Humphrey visual fiels in "worst eye" attributable to central scotoma or "worst eye" visual acuity of 20/200 or worse attributable to primary open-angle glaucoma. "Best eye" may be any stage.

defect type (generalized, mixed, or localized), defined by the intersection of the two values. A-special software is also available for an automated classification of defects.

In the last eight years some other systems have been introduced, including the University of São Paulo Glaucoma Visual Field Staging System (USP-GVFSS), proposed by Susanna and Vessani in 2009,[173] and the Modified Glaucoma Staging System, by Hirashawa *et al.*[174]

The USP-GVFSS uses the Humphrey Visual Field Index (VFI) and the pattern

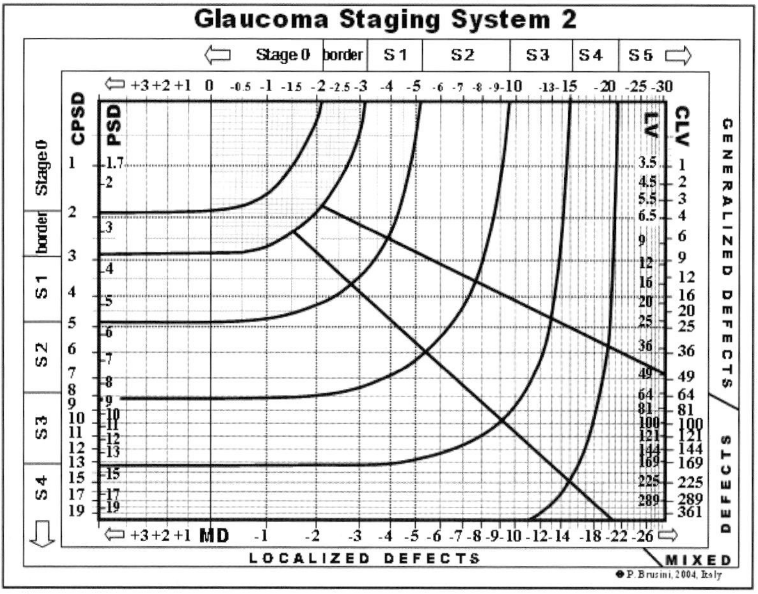

Fig. 5. The Glaucoma Staging System (GSS) version 2.

deviation map in order to characterize the functional loss into three stages (early, moderate and severe VF defect). The abnormality criteria for defining a visual field defect are the same as previously proposed by H-A-P (2). The location of visual field defects (outside or inside the central 10 degrees), the involvement of one or both hemifields, and the connection of defects with the blind spot are also taken into consideration (Fig. 6).

The Modified GSS classifies glaucomatous visual field defects into six stages based on the VFI value only (stage 1 = or > 82%; stage 2 ranging from 63% and 81%; stage 3 ranging from 43% and 62%; stage 4 ranging from 23% and 42%; stage 5 = or < 22%).

Considering the large number of staging methods proposed, the choice regarding which method is best naturally depends on the purpose it intends to serve: quick and easy in a routine clinical setting, standardized and precise in scientific multicenter research studies. Two studies have recently faced this topic: (1) Hamzah JC *et al.*[175] evaluated 33 different staging methods taking into consideration several parameters shown in Table 5, where the five systems with the highest score are compared; (2) Ng *et al.*[176] reported a comparison among the AGIS scoring system, the Mills *et al.* staging system[170] and the GSS 2 (called here eGSS). The authors conclude that "*Of the systems examined in this study, eGSS may be the better choice for its ease of use for both clinicians and researcher.*"

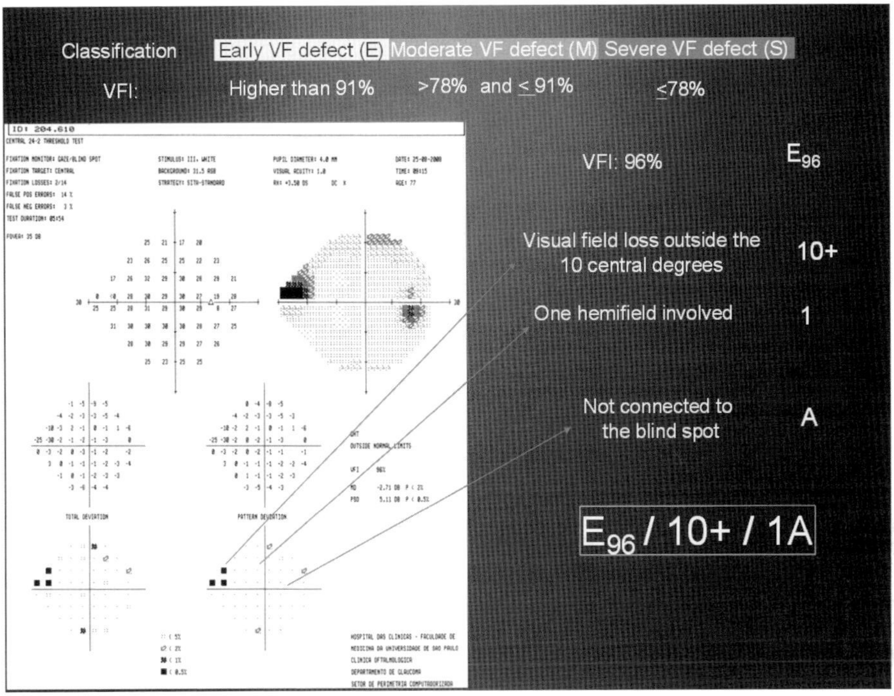

Fig. 6. University of São Paulo Glaucoma Visual Field Staging System.

Of course, no method currently used is perfect. Moreover, one must also keep in mind that perimetry, in itself, is a subjective psychophysical testing method, and thus any classification system that is based on this type of data can never be completely accurate and reproducible.

Table 6, modified from the *Survey Ophthalmology* review previously cited1 by updating by adding new staging systems, can be used as a practical and easy guide to help in the decision making process as to what method is best suited for different needs. The table ranks some of the currently used methods according to the following headings: (1) Name of the staging system; (2) Number of stages utilized; (3) Diagnostic ability for (a) detecting glaucoma defects; (b) defining severity staging; (c) defect type characterization; (d) progression monitoring; (e) disability severity assessment; (4) User-friendliness; (5) Standardization; (6) Widespread use; and (7) Number of references found in literature (PubMed source).

Binocular visual field examination has also sometimes been used in order to weight the amount of functional loss. Gandolfo *et al.* attempted to quantify the amount of visual field loss for medico-legal and insurance purposes.[177] The method uses 100 points, in which the areas located centrally and inferiorly are given greater importance. Binocular visual fields can be scored and quantified with a custom test ('Visual field percent' or VF%) using Humphrey perimeters. The score is based on one hundred tested points within 60 degrees of the visual field using a three-zone screening strategy. The total number of points with a relative or absolute defect are considered in the final score calculation. This method is currently being used in Italy to assess disability caused by visual field constrictions.

Other published papers on the same topic are cited in the references 178-180.

In conclusion, a widespread standardized classification method to stage glaucomatous severity and defect type could be advantageous in both the field of research and in daily clinical practice, and thus emphasis should be placed in achieving this goal and standardizing these procedures on an international level.

Table 5. The five visual field staging systems with the highest score assessed by the quality assessment tool.

Visual Field Stageing System (VFSS)	**Brusini GSS2 (1996&2006)**	**CIGTS VFSS (1998)**	**MD VFSS**	**AGIS VFSS (1994)**	**OCTOSMART (1990)**
Spectrum of glaucoma covered	3	2	2	3	3
Influenced by ocular co-morbidities	2	1	1	1	1
Staging of one or both eyes	1	2	1	1	1
Comprehensible	3	3	3	3	3
Inter-observer reliability	2	3	3	3	3
Test reset reliability	2	3	0	3	1
Responsiveness	3	2	2	3	3
Time to stage	3	3	3	2	3
Available format	2	2	3	2	3
Training needed	2	3	3	1	2
Level of expertise	3	3	3	3	3
Adaptability	3	1	3	1	1
Total score	29	28	27	26	26

57. Lachenmayr BJ, Kojetinsky S, Ostermaier N, et al. The different effects of aging on normal sensitivity in flicker and light-sense perimetry. IOVS 1994;35: 2741-2748.
58. Ramachandran VS, Rogers-Ramachandran D. Phantom Contours: A New Class of Visual Patterns that Selectively Activates the Magnocellular Pathway in Man. Bull Psychonom Soc 1991;29:391.
59. Quaid PT, Simpson TL, Flanagan JG. Frequency doubling illusion: detection vs. form resolution. Optom Vis Sci 2005;8(2):36-42.
60. Goren D, Flanagan JG. Is flicker-defined form (FDF) dependent on the contour? J Vis 2008;8:15.1-15.
61. Horn FK, Kremers J, Mardin CY, et al. Flicker-defined form perimetry in glaucoma patients. Graefes Arch Clin Exp Ophthalmol 2015;253(3):447-455.
62. Lamparter J, Schulze A, Schuff AC, et al. Learning curve and fatigue effect of flicker defined form perimetry. Am J Ophthalmol 2011;151(6):1057-1064.
63. Hasler S, Stürmer J. First experience with the Heidelberg Edge Perimeter® on patients with ocular hypertension and preperimetric glaucoma. Klin Monatsbl Augenheilkd 2012;229(4):319-322.
64. Reznicek L, Lamparter J, Vogel M, Kampik A, Hirneiß C. Flicker defined form perimetry in glaucoma suspects with normal achromatic visual fields. Curr Eye Res 2015;40(7):683-689.
65. Ichhpujani P, Lo DC, Cvintal V, et al. Flicker defined form, standard perimetry and Heidelberg retinal tomography: Structure-function relationships. Can J Ophthalmol 2015;50(4):290-296.
66. Horn FK, Scharch V, Mardin CY, Lämmer R, Kremers J. Comparison of frequency doubling and flicker defined form perimetry in early glaucoma. Graefes Arch Clin Exp Ophthalmol 2016;254(5):937-946.
67. Nowomiejska K, Vonthein R, Paetzold J, et al. Comparison between semi-automated kinetic perimetry and conventional Goldmann manual kinetic perimetry in advanced visual field loss. Ophthalmology 2005;112(8):1343-1354.
68. Nevalainen J, Paetzold J, Krapp E, et al. The use of semi-automated kinetic perimetry (SKP) to monitor advanced glaucomatous visual field loss. Graefes Arch Clin Exp Ophthalmol 2008;246(9):1331-1339.
69. Nowomiejska K, Wrobel-Dudzinska D, Ksiazek K, et al. Semi-automated kinetic perimetry provides additional information to static automated perimetry in the assessment of the remaining visual field in end-stage glaucoma. Ophthalmic Physiol Opt 2015;35(2):147-154.
70. Wilscher S, Wabbels B, Lorenz B. Feasibility and outcome of automated kinetic perimetry in children. Graefes Arch Clin Exp Ophthalmol 2010;248(10):1493-1500.
71. Walters BC, Rahi JS, Cumberland PM. Perimetry in children: survey of current practices in the United Kingdom and Ireland. Ophthalmic Epidemiol 2012;19(6):358-363.
72. Patel DE, Cumberland PM, Walters BC, Russell-Eggitt I, Rahi JS; OPTIC study group. Study of Optimal Perimetric Testing in Children (OPTIC): Feasibility, Reliability and Repeatability of Perimetry in Children. PLoS One 201519;10(6):e0130895.
73. Patel DE, Cumberland PM, Walters BC, Russell-Eggitt I, Cortina-Borja. Study of Optimal Perimetric Testing In Children (OPTIC): Normative Visual Field Values in Children. Ophthalmology 2015;122(8):1711-1717.
74. Stewart WC, Shields MB, Ollie AR. Peripheral visual field testing by automated kinetic perimetry in glaucoma. Arch Ophthalmol 1988;106(2):202-206.
75. Miller KN, Shields MB, Ollie AR. Automated kinetic perimetry with two peripheral isopters in glaucoma. Arch Ophthalmol 1989;107(9):1316-1320.

76. Stewart WC, Shields MB. The peripheral visual field in glaucoma: re-evaluation in the age of automated perimetry. Surv Ophthalmol 1991;36(1):59-69.
77. Stewart WC. Static versus kinetic testing in the nasal peripheral field in patients with glaucoma. Acta Ophthalmol (Copenh) 1992;70(1):79-84.
78. Ballon BJ, Echelman DA, Shields MB, Ollie AR. Peripheral visual field testing in glaucoma by automated kinetic perimetry with the Humphrey Field Analyzer. Arch Ophthalmol 1992;110(12):1730-1732.
79. McLean IM, Mueller E, Buttery RG, Mackey DA. Visual field assessment and the Austroads driving standard. Clin Experiment Ophthalmol 2002;30(1):3-7.
80. Schiefer U, Nowomiejska K, Krapp E, Pätzold J, Johnson CA. K-Train -- a computer-based, interactive training program with an incorporated certification system for practicing kinetic perimetry: evaluation of acceptance and success rate. Graefes Arch Clin Exp Ophthalmol 2006;244(10):1300-1309.
81. Ramirez AM, Chaya CJ, Gordon LK, Giaconi JA. A comparison of semi-automated versus manual Goldmann kinetic perimetry in patients with visually significant glaucoma. J Glaucoma 2008;17(2):111-117.
82. Rowe FJ, Rowlands A. Comparison of diagnostic accuracy between Octopus 900 and Goldmann kinetic visual fields. Biomed Res Int 2014;2014:214829.
83. Gandolfo E. Stato-kinetic dissociation in subjects with normal and abnormal visual fields. Eur J Ophthalmol 1996;6(4):408-414.
84. Schiller J, Paetzold J, Vonthein R, et al. Quantification of stato-kinetic dissociation by semi-automated perimetry. Vision Res 2006;46(1-2):117-128.
85. Dolderer J, Vonthein R, Johnson CA, Schiefer U, Hart W. Scotoma mapping by semi-automated kinetic perimetry: the effects of stimulus properties and the speed of subjects' responses. Acta Ophthalmol Scand 2006;84(3):338-344.
86. Nowomiejska K, Vonthein R, Paetzold J, et al. Reaction time during semi-automated kinetic perimetry (SKP) in patients with advanced visual field loss. Acta Ophthalmol 2010;88(1):65-69.
87. Wakayama A, Matsumoto C, Ohmure K, Inase M, Shimomura Y. Influence of target size and eccentricity on binocular summation of reaction time in kinetic perimetry. Vision Res 2011;51(1):174-178.
88. Nowomiejska K, Brzozowska A, Zarnowski T, et al. Variability in isopter position and fatigue during semi-automated kinetic perimetry. Ophthalmologica 2012;227(3):166-172.
89. Hirasawa K, Shoji N, Okada A, Takano K, Tomioka S. Evaluation of stimulus velocity in automated kinetic perimetry in young healthy participants. Vision Res 2014;98:83-88.
90. Hirasawa K, Shoji N. Learning effect and repeatability of automated kinetic perimetry in healthy participants. Curr Eye Res 2014;39(9):928-937.
91. Hirasawa K, Shoji N, Kobashi C, Yamanashi A. Effects of mydriasis and miosis on kinetic perimetry findings in normal participants. Graefes Arch Clin Exp Ophthalmol 2015;253(8):1341-1346.
92. Hirasawa K, Shoji N, Isono K, Tsuchiya M. Effects of different levels of intraocular stray light on kinetic perimetry findings. PLoS One 2015;10(5):e0127159.
93. Hirasawa K, Shoji N. Effect of Optical Defocus on the Kinetic Perimetry in Young Myopic Participants. Curr Eye Res 2015;40(8):847-852.
94. Schiefer U, Strasburger H, Becker ST, et al. Reaction time in automated kinetic perimetry: effects of stimulus luminance, eccentricity, and movement direction. Vision Res 2001;41(16):2157-

2164.
95. Becker ST, Vonthein R, Volpe NJ, Schiefer U. F actors influencing reaction time during automated kinetic perimetry on the Tubingen computer campimeter. Invest Ophthalmol Vis Sci 2005;46(7):2633-2638.
96. Vonthein R, Rauscher S, Paetzold J, et al. The normal age-corrected and reaction time-corrected isopter derived by semi-automated kinetic perimetry. Ophthalmology 2007;114(6):1065-1072.
97. Shapiro LR, Johnson CA. Quantitative evaluation of manual kinetic perimetry using computer simulation. Appl Opt 1990;29(10):1445-1450.
98. Hashimoto S, Matsumoto C, Okuyama S, et al. Development of a new fully automated kinetic algorithm (program k) for detection of glaucomatous visual field loss. Invest Ophthalmol Vis Sci 2015;56(3):2092-2099.
99. Bedwell CH. Recent developments in investigations of visual fields. Am J Optom Physiol Opt 1978;55(10):681-699.
100. Pineles SL, Volpe NJ, Miller-Ellis E, et al. Automated combined kinetic and static perimetry: an alternative to standard perimetry in patients with neuro-ophthalmic disease and glaucoma. Arch Ophthalmol 2006;124(3):363-369.
101. Westcott MC, Fitzke FW, Hitchings RA. Abnormal motion displacement thresholds are associated with fine scale luminance sensitivity loss in glaucoma. Vision Research 1998;38:3171-3180.
102. Westcott MC, Fitzke FW, Viswanathan AC, Hitchings RA. Response time prolongation for a motion stimulus in patients with glaucoma and its relationship with elevation of the motion threshold. J Glaucoma 2000;9:289-295.
103. Baez KA, McNaught AI, Dowler JG, et al. Motion detection threshold and field progression in normal tension glaucoma. Br J Ophthalmol 1995;79(2):125-128.
104. Wall M. Ketoff KM. Random dot motion perimetry in patients with glaucoma and in normal subjects. Am J Ophthalmol 1995;120:587-596.
105. Wall M, Jennisch CS. Random dot motion stimuli are more sensitive than light stimuli for detection of visual field loss in ocular hypertension patients. Optom Vis Sci 1999;76:550-557.
106. Wall M, Jennisch CS, Munden PM. Motion perimetry identifies nerve fiber bundlelike defects in ocular hypertension. Arch Ophthalmol 1997;115:26-33.
107. Gonzalez-Hernandez M, Fernandez-Vidal A, Garcia-Feijoo J, Gonzalez de la Rosa M. Combined spatial resolution and contrast perimetry in normal subjects. In: Wall M, Millam RP (Eds.), Perimetry Update 2000/2001, pp. 109-114. The Hague: Kugler Publications 2001.
108. Bergin C, Redmond T, Nathwani N, et al. The effect of induced intraocular straylight on perimetric tests. Invest Ophthalmol Vis Sci 2011;52(6):3676-3682.
109. Ong EL, Zheng Y, Aung T, et al. Performance of the Moorfields motion displacement test for identifying eyes with glaucoma. Ophthalmology 2014;121:88-92.
110. Dabasia PL, Fidalgo BR, Edgar DF, Garway-Heath DF, Lawrenson JG. Diagnostic Accuracy of Technologies for Glaucoma Case-Finding in a Community Setting. Ophthalmology 2015;122:2407-2415.
111. Gonzalez de la Rosa M, Gonzalez-Hernandez M. Pulsar perimetry. A review and new results. Ophthalmologe 2013;110(2):107-115.
112. González de la Rosa, M, González-Hernández M, García-Feijoo J, Sánchez Méndez M, García-Sánchez J. Comparing the ranges of defect measured with standard white on white and Pulsar perimetries. Arch Soc Esp Oftalmol 2011;86(4):113-117.
113. Gonzalez-Hernandez M, de la Rosa MG, de la Vega RR, Hernandez-Vidal A. Long-term fluc-

tuation of standard automatic perimetry, pulsar perimetry and frequency-doubling technology in early glaucoma diagnosis. Ophthalmic Res 2007;39(6):338-343.

114. Salvetat ML, Zeppieri M, Parisi L, et al. Learning effect and test-retest variability of pulsar perimetry. J Glaucoma 2013;22(3):230-237.

115. González-Hernández M, Abreu A, Sánchez M, González de la Rosa M. Combined spatial, contrast and temporal function perimetry in early glaucoma and ocular hypertension. In: Henson DB, Wall M (Eds.), Perimetry Update 2002/2003, p. 247. Amsterdam: Kugler Publications 2004.

116. Fernández-Vidal AM, García-Feijoo J, García-Sánchez J. Pulsar perimetry: a new procedure for early glaucoma evaluation. In: Henson D, Wall M (Eds.), Perimetry Update 2002/2003, pp. 199-205. Amsterdam: Kugler Pub 2004.

117. Fernández-Vidal A, García Feijoo J, González-Hernández M, González de la Rosa M, García Sánchez J. Primeros hallazgos con perimetría Pulsar en pacientes hipertensos oculares. Arch Soc Esp Oftalmol 2002;77:321-326.

118. González-Hernández M, García-Feijoo J, Sánchez Méndez M, González de la Rosa M. Combined spatial, contrast and temporal functions perimetry in mild glaucoma and ocular hipertensión. Eur J Ophthalmol 2004;14:514-522.

119. González de la Rosa M, Méndez Hernández C, García Feijoo J, et al. TOP strategy and Pulsar T30W perimetry in glaucomaearly diagnosis. In: Reece SM (Ed.), Focus on Glaucoma Research, pp. 117-172. New York: Nova Science Publishers Inc. 2005.

120. Salvetat ML, Zeppieri M, Tosoni C, Parisi L, Brusini P. Non-conventional perimetric methods in the detection of early glaucomatous functional damage. Eye (Lond) 2010;24(5):835-842.

121. Frisén L. New, sensitive window on abnormal spatial vision: rarebit probing. Vis Res 2002;42:1931-1939.

122. Brusini P, Salvetat ML, Parisi L, Zeppieri M. Probing glaucoma visual damage by rarebit perimetry. British Journal of Ophthalmology 2005;89:180-184.

123. Frisén L. Performance of a rapid rarebit central-vision test with optic neuropathies. Optom Vis Sci 2012;89:1192-1195.

124. Hackett DA, Anderson AJ. Determining mechanisms of visual loss in glaucoma using Rarebit perimetry. Optom Vis Sci 2011;88:48-55.

125. Winther C, Frisén L. New rarebit vision test captures macular deficits hidden to acuity tests. Acta Ophthalmologica 2015;93:481-485.

126. Wall M, Doyle CK, Eden T, Zamba KD, Johnson CA. Size threshold perimetry performs as well as conventional automated perimetry with sizes III, V, and VI for glaucomatous detection loss. IOVS 2013;54:3975-3983.

127. Gordon-Bennett PS, Ioannidis AS, Papageorgiou K, Andreou PS. A survey of investigations used for the management of glaucoma in hospital service in the United Kingdom. Eye (Lond) 2008;22(11):1410-1418.

128. Myint J, Edgar DF, Kotecha A, Murdoch IE, Lawrenson JG. A national survey of diagnostic tests reported by UK community optometrists for the detection of chronic open angle glaucoma. Ophthalmic Physiol Opt 2011;31(4):353-359. doi: 10.1111/j.1475-1313.2011.00844.x.

129. Garway-Heath DF, Crabb DP, Bunce C, et al. Latanoprost for open-angle glaucoma (UKGTS): a randomised, multicentre, placebo-controlled trial. Lancet 2015;4;385(9975):1295-1304.

130. Heijl A, Bengtsson B, Chauhan BC,et al. A comparison of visual field progression criteria of 3 major glaucoma trials in early manifest glaucoma trial patients. Ophthalmology 2008;115(9):1557-1565.

131. Van der Schoot J, et al. The ability of short-wavelength automated perimetry to predict conversion to glaucoma. Ophthalmology 2010;117(1):30-34.
132. Johnson CA. Recent developments in automated perimetry in glaucoma diagnosis and management. Curr Opin Ophthalmol 2002;13(2):77-84.
133. Xin D, Greenstein VC, Ritch R, Liebmann JM, De Moraes CG, Hood DC. A comparison of functional and structural measures for identifying progression of glaucoma. Invest Ophthalmol Vis Sci 2011;52(1):519-526.
134. Fan X, Wu LL, Ma ZZ, Xiao GG, Liu F Jr. Usefulness of frequency-doubling technology for perimetrically normal eyes of open-angle glaucoma patients with unilateral field loss. Ophthalmology 2010;117(8):1530-1537.
135. Haymes SA, Hutchison DM, McCormick TA, et al. Glaucomatous visual field progression with frequency-doubling technology and standard automated perimetry in a longitudinal prospective study. Invest Ophthalmol Vis Sci 2005;46(2):547-554.
136. Fitzke FW. Clinical psychophysics. Eye 1988;2 Suppl:S233-241.
137. Verdon-Roe GM, Westcott MC, Viswanathan AC, Fitzke FW, Garway-Heath DF. Exploration of the psychophysics of a motion displacement hyperacuity stimulus. Invest Ophthalmol Vis Sci 2006;47(11):4847-4855.
138. Demirel S, De Moraes CGV, Gardiner SK, et al.; the Ocular Hypertension Treatment Study Group. Rate of Visual Field Change in the Ocular Hypertension Treatment Study. Invest Ophthalmol Vis Sci 2012;53(1):224-227.
139. Artes PH, Chauhan BC, Keltner JL, et al.; the Ocular Hypertension Treatment Study Group. Longitudinal and Cross-sectional Analyses of Visual Field Progression in Participants of the Ocular Hypertension Treatment Study. Arch Ophthalmol 2010;128(12):1528-1532.
140. Baez KA, McNaught AI, Dowler JG, Poinoosawmy D, Fitzke FW, Hitchings RA Motion detection threshold and field progression in normal tension glaucoma. Br J Ophthalmol 1995;79(2):125-128.
141. Cho HK, Suh W, Kee C. Visual and structural prognosis of the untreated fellow eyes of unilateral normal tension glaucoma patients. Graefes Arch Clin Exp Ophthalmol 2015;253(9):1547-1555.
142. Membrey WL, Poinoosawmy DP, Bunce C, Fitzke FW, Hitchings RA. Comparison of visual field progression in patients with normal pressure glaucoma between eyes with and without visual field loss that threatens fixation. Br J Ophthalmol 2000; 84(10):1154-1158.
143. Strouthidis NG, Scott A, Peter NM, Garway-Heath DF. Optic Disc and Visual Field Progression in Ocular Hypertensive Subjects: Detection Rates, Specificity, and Agreement'. Invest Ophthalmol Vis Sci 2006;47(7):2904-2910.
144. Bach M, Hoffmann MB. Update on the pattern electroretinogram in glaucoma. Optom Vis Sci 2008;85:386-395.
145. Bach M, Poloschek CM. Electrophysiology and glaucoma: current status and future chal-lenges. Cell Tissue Res 2013;353:287-296.
146. Ventura LM, Porciatti V. Pattern electroretinogram in glaucoma. Curr Opin Ophthalmol 2006;17:196-202.
147. Graham SL, Fortune B. Electrophysiology in glaucoma assessment. In: Shaarawy TM, Sherwood MB, Hitchings RA, Crowston JG (Eds.), Glaucoma, 2nd Edi-tion, pp. 149-168. London: Elsevier 2015.
148. Porciatti V. Electrophysiological assessment of retinal ganglion cell function. Exp Eye Res 2015;141:164-170.

149. Wilsey LJ, Fortune B. Electroretinography in glaucoma diagnosis. Curr Opin Ophthalmol 2016;27(2):118-124.
150. Banitt MR, Ventura LM, Feuer WJ, et al. Progressive loss of retinal ganglion cell function precedes structural loss by several years in glaucoma suspects. Invest Ophthalmol Vis Sci 2013;54:2346-2352.
151. Bode SF, Jehle T, Bach M. Pattern electroretinogram in glaucoma suspects: new findings from a longitudinal study. Invest Ophthalmol Vis Sci 2011;52:4300-4306.
152. Hood DC, Xu L, Thienprasiddhi P, et al. The pattern electroretinogram in glaucoma patients with confirmed visual field deficits. Invest Ophthalmol Vis Sci 2005;46:2411-2418.
153. Viswanathan S, Frishman LJ, Robson JG, et al. The photopic negative response of the macaque electroretinogram: reduction by experimental glaucoma. Invest Ophthalmol Vis Sci 1999;40:1124-1136.
154. Viswanathan S, Frishman LJ, Robson JG, Walters JW. The photopic negative response of the flash electroretinogram in primary open angle glaucoma. Invest Ophthalmol Vis Sci 2001;42:514-522.
155. Machida S. Clinical applications of the photopic negative response to optic nerve and retinal diseases. J Ophthalmol 2012;2012:397178.
156. Niyadurupola N, Luu CD, Nguyen DQ, et al. Intraocular pressure lowering is associated with an increase in the photopic negative response (PhNR) amplitude in glaucoma and ocular hypertensive eyes. Invest Ophthalmol Vis Sci 2013;54:1913-1919.
157. Machida S, Kaneko M, Kurosaka D. Regional variations in correlation between photopic negative response of focal electoretinograms and ganglion cell complex in glaucoma. Curr Eye Res 2015;40:439-449.
158. Hood DC, Greenstein VC. Multifocal VEP and ganglion cell damage: applications and limitations for the study of glaucoma. Prog Retin Eye Res 2003;22:201-251.
159. Klistorner AI, Graham SL, Grigg JR, Billson FA. Multifocal topographic visual evoked potential: improving objective detection of local visual field defects. Invest Ophthalmol Vis Sci 1998;39:937-950.
160. Graham SL, Klistorner AI, Goldberg I. Clinical application of objective perimetry using multifocal visual evoked potentials in glaucoma practice. Arch Ophthalmol 2005;123:729-739.
161. Fortune B, Demirel S, Zhang X, et al. Comparing multifocal VEP and standard automated perimetry in high-risk ocular hypertension and early glaucoma. Invest Ophthalmol Vis Sci 2007;48:1173-1180.
162. De Moraes CG, Liebmann JM, Ritch R, Hood DC. Clinical use of multifocal visual-evoked potentials in a glaucoma practice: a prospective study. Doc Ophthalmol 2012;125:1-9.
163. Hood DC, Ritch R. Other tests in glaucoma: multifocal visual evoked potential. In: Giaconi JA, Law SK, Coleman AL, Caprioli J. (Eds.), Pearls of Glaucoma Management, pp. 175-181. Berlin/Heidelberg: Springer 2010.
164. Klistorner A, Graham SL. Objective perimetry in glaucoma. Ophthalmology 2000;107:2283-2299.
165. Caprioli J, Sears M, Spaeth GL. Comparison of visual field defects in normal-tension glaucoma and high-tension glaucoma. Am J Ophthalmol 1986;102:402-404.
166. Brusini P, Johnson CA. Staging functional damage in glaucoma: review of different classification methods. Surv Ophthalmol 2007;52:156-179.
167. Hodapp E, Parrish II RK, Anderson DR. Clinical decisions in glaucoma, pp 52-61. St. Louis: The C.V. Mosby Comp 1993.

168. The Advanced Glaucoma Intervention Study Investigators. Advanced glaucoma intervention study. Visual field test scoring and reliability. Ophthalmology 1994;101:1445-1455.
169. Musch D, Lichter PR, Guire KE, Standardi CL; for the CIGTS Study Group. The Collaborative Initial Glaucoma Treatment Study. Study design, methods, and baseline characteristics of enrolled patients. Ophthalmology 1999;106:653-662.
170. Mills RP, Budenz DL, Lee PP, et al. Categorizing the stage of glaucoma from pre-diagnosis to end-stage disease. Am J Ophthalmol 2006;141:24-30.
171. Brusini P. Clinical use of a new method for visual field damage classification in glaucoma. Eur J Ophthalmol 1996;6:402-407.
172. Brusini P, Filacorda S. Enhanced glaucoma staging system (GSS 2) for classifying functional damage in glaucoma. J Glaucoma 2006;15:40-46.
173. Susanna R Jr, Vessani RM. Staging glaucoma patient: why and how? Open Ophthalmol J 2009;3:59-64.
174. Hirasawa K, Shoji N, Morita T, Shimizu K. A modified glaucoma staging system based on visual field index. Graefes Arch Clin Exp Ophthalmol 2013;251:2747-2752.
175. Hamzah JC, Ramsay CR, Azuara-Blanco A, Burt JM. Systematic evaluation of visual field staging systems for glaucoma. Poster ARVO, Fort Lauderdale, 1-5 May 2011.
176. Ng M, Sample PA, Pascual JP, et al. Comparison of visual field severity classification system for glaucoma. J Glaucoma 2012;21:551-561.
177. Gandolfo E, Zingirian M, Capris P. A new proposal for classification and quantification of visual disability In: Mills RP, Heijl A (Eds.), Perimetry Update 1990/91, pp. 545-549. Amsterdam/New York: Kugler Publications 1991.
178. Morescalchi F, Gandolfo E, Gandolfo F, Quaranta L, Capris P. A new scoring program for quantification of the binocular visual field. In: Henson DB, Wall M (Eds.), Perimetry Update 2002/2003, pp. 21-27. The Hague, The Netherlands: Kugler Publications 2004.
179. McGwin G Jr, Xie A, Mays A, et al. Visual field defects and the risk of motor vehicle collisions among patients with glaucoma. Invest Ophthalmol Vis Sci 2005;46:4437-4441.
180. Hu S, Smith ND, Saunders LJ, Crabb DP. Patterns of Binocular Visual Field Loss Derived from Large-Scale Patient Data from Glaucoma Clinics. Ophthalmology 2015;122(12):2399-2406.
181. Quigley HA, Broman AT. The number of people with glaucoma worldwide in 2010 and 2020. Br J Ophthalmol 2006;90:243-254.
182. Tham Y-C, Li X, Wong TY, et al. Global prevalence of glaucoma and projections of glaucoma burden through 2040. Ophthalmology 2014;121:2081-2090.
183. Saunders LJ, Russell RA, Crabb DP. Practical landmarks for visual field disability in glaucoma. Br J Ophthalmol 2012;96(9):1185-1189.
184. Owsley C, Wood JM, McGwin G Jr. A roadmap for interpreting the literature on vision and driving. Surv Ophthalmol 2015;60(3):250-262
185. Gutierrez P, Wilson MR, Johnson C, et al. Influence of glaucomatous visual field loss on health-related quality of life. Arch Ophthalmol 1997;115:777-784.
186. Sherwood MB, Garcia-Siekavizza A, Meltzer MI, et al. Glaucoma's impact on quality of life and its relation to clinical indicators. A pilot study. Ophthalmology 1998;105:561-566.
187. Janz NK, Wren PA, Lichter PR, et al. Quality of life in newly diagnosed glaucoma patients: The collaborative initial glaucoma treatment study. Ophthalmology 2001;108(5):887-897.
188. Sumi I, Shirato S, Matsumoto S, Araie M. The relationship between visual disability and visual field in patients with glaucoma. Ophthalmology 2003;110:332-339.
189. Vandenbroeck S, De Geest S, Zeyen T, Stalmans I, Dobbels F. Patient-reported outcomes

(PRO's) in glaucoma: a systematic review. Eye 2011;25:555-577.

190. American Academy of Ophthalmology Preferred Practice Patterns Glaucoma Panel. Primary Open-Angle Glaucoma. San Francisco: American Academy of Ophthalmology 2000.

191. Ramulu PY, Maul E, Hochberg C, et al. Real-world assessment of physical activity in glaucoma using an accelerometer. Ophthalmology 2012;119:1155-1166.

192. Kong XM, Zhu WQ, Hong JX, Sun XH. Is glaucoma comprehension associated with psychological disturbance and vision-related quality of life for patients with glaucoma? A cross-sectional study. BMJ Open 2014.

193. Qiu M, Wang SY, Singh K, Lin SC. Association between visual field defects and quality of life in the United states. Ophthalmology 2014;121:733-740.

194. McKean-Cowdin R, Wang Y, Wu J, Zen SP, Varma R; Los Angeles Latino Eye Study Group. Impact of visual field loss on health-related quality of life in glaucoma. Ophthalmology 2008;115:941-948.

195. Nguyen AM, van Landingham SW, Massof RW, Rubin GS, Ramulu PY. Reading ability and reading engagement in older adults with glaucoma. Invest Ophthalmol Vis Sci 2014;55:5284-5290.

196. Ramulu PY, Swenor BK, Jefferys JL, Friedman DS, Rubin GS. Difficulty with out-loud and silent reading in glaucoma. Invest Ophthalmol Vis Sci 2013;54:666-672.

197. Floriani I, Quaranta L, Rulli E et al. Health-related quality of life in patients with primary open-angle glaucoma. An Italian multicenter observational study. Acta Ophthalmol 2015 Nov 19. doi: 10.1111/aos.12890. [Epub ahead of print]

198. Peters D, Heijl A, Brenner L, Bengtsson B. Visual impairment and vision-related quality of life in the Early Manifest Glaucoma Trial after 20 years of follow-up. Acta Ophthalmol 2015;93:745-752.

199. Yuki K, Tanabe S, Kouyama K, et al. The association between visual field defects severity and fear of falling in primary open-angle glaucoma. Invest Ophthalmol Vis Sci 2013;54:7739-7745.

200. Gothwal VK, Reddy SP, Bharani S, et al. Impact of glaucoma on visual functioning in Indians. Invest Ophthalmol Vis Sci 2012;53:6081-6092.

201. Burton R, Crabb DP, Smith ND, Glen FC, Garway-Heath DF. Glaucoma and Reading: Exploring the effects of contrast lowering of text. Optometry Vsi Sci 2012;89:1282-1287.

202. Onakoya AO, Mbadugha CA, Aribaba OT, Ibidapo OO. Quality of life of primary open angle glaucoma patients in Lagos, Nigeria; clinical and sociodemographic correlates. J Glaucoma 2012;21:287-295.

203. Ramulu PY, van Landingham SW, Massof RW, et al. Fear of falling and visual field loss from glaucoma. Ophthalmology 2012;119:135208.

204. Okamoto M, Sugisaki K, Murata H, et al. Impact of better and worse eye damage on quality of life in advanced glaucoma. Scientific Reports 4, Article number:4144(2014) doi:10.1038.

205. Arora KS, Boland MV, Friedman DS, et al. Relationship between better-eye and integrated visual field mean deviation and visual disability. Ophthalmology 2013;2010:2476-2484.

206. Sawada H, Yoshino T, Fukuchi T, Abe H. Assessment of the vision-specific quality of life using clustered visual field in glaucoma patients. J Glaucoma 2014;23:81-87.

207. Kulkarni KM, Mayer R, Lorenzana LL, Myers SS, Spaeth GL. Visual field staging systems in glaucoma and the activities of daily living. Am J Ophthalmol 2012;154:445-451.

208. Magacho L, Lima FE, Nery AC, et al. Quality of life in glaucoma patients: regression analysis and correlation with possible modifiers. Ophthalmic Epidemiol 2004;11:263-270.

209. Gothwal VK, Bagga DK, Rao HO, et al. Is utility-based quality of life in adults affected by

glaucoma? Invest Ophthalmol Vis Sci 2014;55:1361-1369.
210. Hirooka K, Sato S, Nitta E, Tsujikawa A. The relationship between vision-related quality of life and visual function in glaucoma patients. J Glaucoma 2016.;25(6):505-509
211. Murata H, Hirasawa H, Aoyama Y, et al. Identifying areas of the visual field important for quality of life in patients with glaucoma. PLos One 8,e58695 10.1371/journal.pone.0058695(2013).
212. Esterman B. functional scoring of the binocular field. Ophthalmology 1982;89:1226-1234.
213. Mills RP, Drance SM. Easterman disability rating in severe glaucoma. Ophthalmology 1986;93:371-378.
214. Crabb DP, Viswanathan AC, McNaught AI, et al. Simulating binocular visual field status in glaucoma. Br J Ophthalmol 1998;82:1236-1241.
215. Jampel HD, Friedman DS, Quigley HA, Miller A. correlation of the binocular visual field with patient assessment of vision. Invest Ophthalmol Vis Sci 2002;43:1059-1067.
216. Nelson-Quigg JM, Cello K, Johnson CA. Predicting binocular visual field sensitivity from monocular visual field results. Invest Ophthalmol Vis Sci 2000;41:3312-3321.
217. Asaoka R, Crabb DP, Yamashita T, et al. Patients have two eyes!: binocular versus better eye visual field indices. Invest Ophthalmol Vis Sci 2011;52(9):7007-7011.
218. Black AA, Wood JM, Lovie-Kitchin JE. Inferior field loss increases rate of falls in older adults with glaucoma. Optom Vis Sci 2011;88:1275-1282.
219. Van Gestel A, Weber CA, Beckers HJ et al. The relationship between visual field loss and health-related quality of life. Eye 2010;24:1759-69.
220. Cheng HC, Guo Cy, Cheng MJ, et al. Patient-reported vision-related quality of life differences between superior and inferior hemifield defects in primary open-angle glaucoma. JAMA Ophthalmol 2015;133:269-75.
221. Takahashi GI, Otori Y, Urashima M, Kuwayama Y. Evaluation of quality of life in Japanese glaucoma patients and its relationship with visual function. Quality of Life Improvement Committee. J Glaucoma. 2016 ;25(3):e150-156.
222. Sun Y, Linc C, Waisbourd M, et al. The impact of visual field clusters on performance-based measures and vision-related quality of life in patients with glaucoma. Am J Ophthalmol 2016;163:45-52
223. Freeman EE, Muñoz B, Rubin G, West SK. Visual field loss increases the risk of falls in older adults: the Salisbury eye evaluation. Invest Ophthalmol Vis Sci 2007;48(10):4445-4450.
224. Suzuki Y, Araie M, Ohashi Y. Sectorization of central 30 degrees visual field in glaucoma. Ophthalmology 1993;100:69-75.
225. Douglas PK, Harris S, Yuille A, et al. Performance comparison of machine-learning algorithms and number of independent components used in fMRI decoding of belief vs. disbelief. Neuroimage 2011;56:544-553.
226. Hirasawa H, Murata H, Mayama C, Araie M, Asaoka R. Evaluation of various machine learning methods to predict vision-related quality of life from visual field data and visual acuity in patients with glaucoma. Br J Ophthalmol 2014;98:1230-1235.
227. Ekici F, Loh R, Waisbourd M, et al. Relationships Between Measures of the Ability to Perform Vision-Related Activities, Vision-Related Quality of Life, and Clinical Findings in Patients With Glaucoma. JAMA Ophthalmol 2015;133(12):1377-1385.
228. Richman J, Lorenzana LL, Lankaranian D, et al. Relationships in glaucoma patients between standard vision tests, quality of life, and ability to perform daily activities. Ophthalmic Epidemiol 2010;17(3):144-151.
229. Freeman EE, Muñoz B, West SK, Jampel HD, Friedman DS. Glaucoma and quality of life: the

270. Lisboa R, Chun YS, Zangwill LM, et al. Association between rates of binocular visual field loss and vision-related quality of life in patients with glaucoma. JAMA Ophthalmol 2013;131:486-494.
271. Gracitelli CP, Abe RY, Tatham AJ, et al. Association between progressive retinal nerve fiber layer loss and longitudinal change in quality of life in glaucoma. JAMA Ophthalmol 2015;133:384-390.
272. Medeiros FA, Cracitelli CPB, Boer ER, et al. Longitudinal changes in quality of life and rates of progressive visual field loss in glaucoma patients. Ophthalmology 2015;122:293-301.
273. Abe RY, Diniz-Filho A, Costa VP, et al. The impact of location of progressive visual field loss on longitudinal changes in quality of life of patients with glaucoma. Ophthalmology 2016;123(3):552-557.
274. Hyman LG, Komaroff E, Heijl A, Bengtsson B, Leske MC; the Early Manifest Glaucoma Trial Group. Treatment and vision-related quality of life in the Early Manifest Glaucoma Trial. Ophthalmology 2005;112:1505-1513.
275. Kerr MN, Patel HY, Chew SSL, et al. Patient satisfaction with topical ocular hypotensives. Clin Exp Ophthalmol 2013;41:27-35.
276. Rossi GC, Tinelli C, Pasinetti GM, Milano G, Bianchi PE. Dry eye syndrome-related quality of life in glaucoma patients. Eur J Ophthalmol 2009;19:572-579.
277. Skalicky, SE, Goldberg I, Mccluskey P. Ocular surface disease and quality of life in patients with glaucoma. Am J Ophthalmol 2012;153:1-9.
278. Actis AG, Rolle T. Ocular surface alterations and topical antiglaucomatous therapy: a review. Open Ophthalmol J 2014;8:67-72.
279. Nordmann J-P, Auzanneau A, Ricard S, Berdeaux G. Vision related quality of life ant topical glaucoma treatment side effects. Health and Quality of Life Outcomes 2003;1:75.
280. Loon SC, Jin J, Goh MJ. The relationship between quality of life and adherence to medication in glaucoma patients in Singapore. J Glaucoma 2015;24:e36-342.
281. Rossi GC, Pasinetti GM, Scudeller L, Raimondi M, Lanteri S, Bianchi PE. Risk factors to develop ocular surface disease in treated glaucoma or ocular hypertension patients. Eur J Ophthalmol 2013;23:296-302.
282. Baudouin C, Renard J-P, Nordmann J-P, et al. Prevalence and risk factors for ocular surface disease among patients treated over the long term for glaucoma or ocular hypertension. Eur J Ophthalmol 2013;23:47-54.
283. Michele I, Serena T, Paolo F, et al. Ocular surface changes in glaucomatous patients treated with and without preservatives beta-blockers. J Ocul Pharmacol Ther 2014;30:476-481.
284. Pinto LA, Vandewalle E, Gerlier L, Stalmans I; The Cosopt UD Switch Study Group. Improvement in glaucoma patient quality of life by therapy switch to preservative-free timolol/dorzolamide fixed combination. Ophthalmologe 2014;231:166-171.
285. Dunker S, Schmucker A, Maier H; The Latanoprost/Timolol Fixed Combination Study Group. Adv Ther 2007;24:376-386.
286. Mathews PM, Ramulu PY, Friedman DS, Utine CA, Akpek EK. Evaluation of ocular surface disease in patients with glaucoma. Ophthalmology 2013;120(11):2241-2248.
287. Janz NK, Wren PA, Lichter PR, et al. The Collaborative Initial Glaucoma Treatment Study. Interim quality of life findings after initial medical or surgical treatment of glaucoma. Ophthalmology 2001;108:1954-1965.
288. Guedes RAP, Guedes VM, Freitas SM, Chaoubah A. Quality of life of medically versus surgically treated glaucoma patients. J Glaucoma 2013;22:369-373.

289. Bailey LA, Okereke OI, Kawachi I, et al. Ophthalmic and glaucoma treatment characteristics associated with changes in health-related quality of life before and after newly diagnosed primary open-angle glaucoma in nurses' health study participants. J Glaucoma 2016;25(3):e220-228.
290. Klink K, Sauer J, Körber NJ, et al. Quality of life following glaucoma surgery: canaloplasty versus trabeculectomy. Clin Ophthalmol 2014;9:7-16.

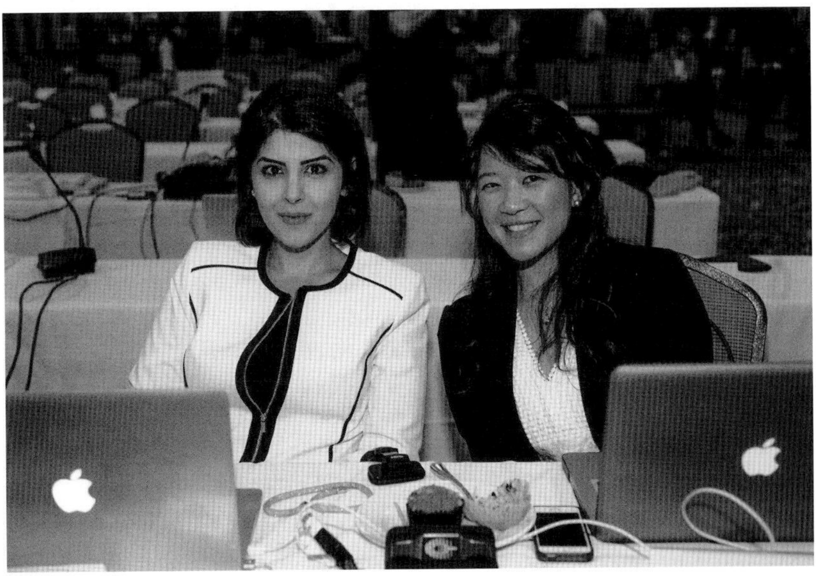

Consensus X recording secretaries: Adeleh Yarmohammadi and Patricia Manlastas

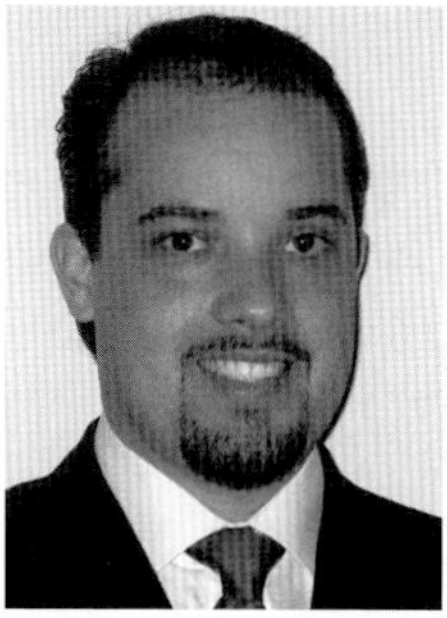

Felipe A. Medeiros

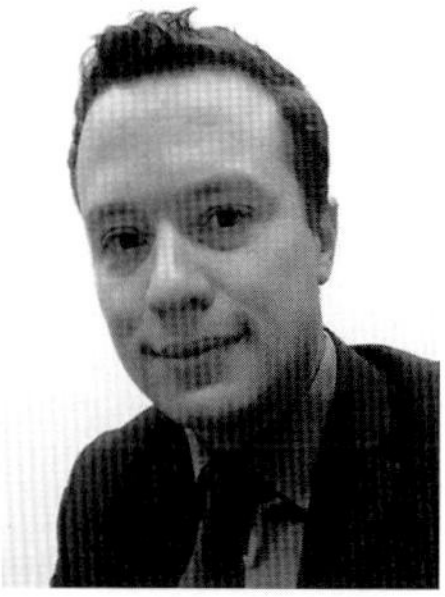

Gustavo De Moreas

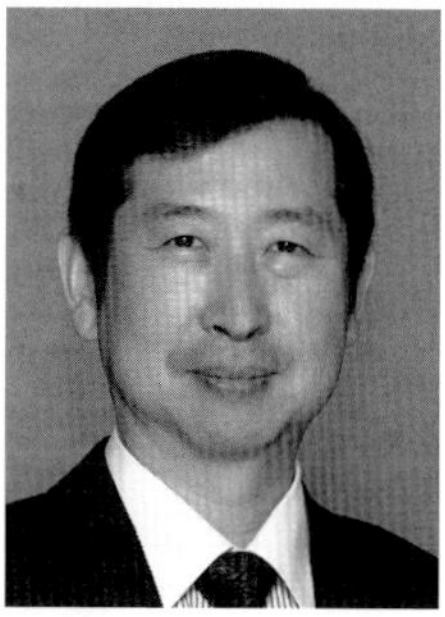

Ki Ho Park

3. STRUCTURE & FUNCTION

Section leader: Felipe A. Medeiros
Section co-leaders: Gustavo De Moraes, Ki Ho Park
Contributors: Makoto Araie, Eytan Blumenthal, Joseph Caprioli, Murray Fingeret, John Flanagan, Christopher Girkin, Donald Hood, Tae-Woo Kim, Miriam Kolko, Catherine Liu, Jose Martinez de la Casa, Allison Maree McKendrick, Kouros Nouri-Mahdavi, Lyne Racette, Harsha Rao, Lisandro Sakata, Andrew Tatham, Christopher Teng

Consensus statements

1. In glaucoma, there is a continuous relationship between standard structural and functional (dB for visual field) measurements, which appears nonlinear with current methods of testing and conventional scaling of metrics.
   Comment: When both are transformed into linear scales, then a linear relationship between structure and function can be observed.
2. Current structural and functional measurement methods show considerable variability.
3. Visual field test locations are spatially related to regions on the optic nerve head, peripapillary retina and macular area.
   Comment: Understanding these spatial relationships can be useful for the diagnosis of glaucoma.
4. With current technology, detection of structural defects generally precedes detectable functional defects in glaucoma patients while functional defects can precede structural defects in some patients.
   Comment: Structural tests based on the comparison to the normative data tend to show a statistically significant glaucomatous change earlier compared to the functional tests because of a greater variability in functional tests.
5. The likelihood of the diagnosis of glaucoma is increased through corroboration of abnormal structural and functional tests.
   Comment: The likelihood of the diagnosis of glaucoma is increased further if there is progressive change or if additional risk factors are present, such as

Diagnosis of Primary Open Angle Glaucoma, pp 91-124
Edited by Robert N. Weinreb, David Garway-Heath, Christopher Leung, Felipe Medeiros, Jeffrey Liebmann

raised intraocular pressure.

6. When available, OCT (or an alternative imaging modality) and disc photographs with acceptable quality at baseline should be performed, against which accurate detection of change can be made.
   Comments: Disc photography is a useful adjunct for detecting hemorrhages and pallor, and also for assessing change compared with future clinical examinations.
   Disc hemorrhages can only be seen on clinical examinations and disc photographs.
7. As yet there is no widely-accepted method of combining the results of structural and functional tests.
   Comment: Several proposed methods for combining structural and/or functional measurements offer advantages over traditional parameters and continue to be investigated.
8. Physicians should be aware of false-positive tests and over-diagnosing glaucoma, which are more likely when using a large number of diagnostic tests.
   Comment: Although using multiple parameters may increase overall diagnostic sensitivity, the chance will also increase of falsely labeling a change significant.

3.1. Structure and function relationship in glaucoma: How is structural damage related to functional loss in glaucoma? Summary of current structure-function models in glaucoma

a. Current proposed models linking structure and function in glaucoma
   - Harwerth *et al.*'s model:[1] VF threshold sensitivity vs. RGC density;
   - The Hood-Kardon model[2] (simple linear model);
   - The 'Hockey-Stick' model: changing slope of SF relationship as a function of eccentricity;
   - Drasdo *et al.*'s model:[3]
     - The bipartite model linking RGC density to VF sensitivity;
     - also addresses the displacement of the RGCs within the central macula as pertains correspondence with the central VF test locations.

b. Factors affecting precision of the structure function relationships
   - Measurement variability for both structural and functional measures;

- Scale of measurements: Linear for structural, logarithmic for functional measures;
- Range of glaucoma severity;
- Non-neural elements of the RNFL, neuroretinal rim or macular measures;
- Relationship between axon number and RNFL thickness;
- Variations in relationship of the disc anatomy versus foveal location: variability in the ONH entry point for a given visual field location: 20-30 degrees variation;
- Averaging dilutes a lot of localized loss; also, the averaging within structure and function is not uniform and some structural regions match wider clusters of VF and vice versa; this includes unevenness of sampling for the 24-2 grid.

c. Other confounding psychophysical factors
  - Ricco's area and spatial summation;
  - Cortical pooling.

d. Macular structure-function relationships: What is different?
e. The RGC count as a unifying link between structure and function.

3.1.1. Introduction

Glaucoma is an optic neuropathy characterized by typical changes on optic nerve head and retinal nerve fiber layer (RNFL). These structural changes usually lead to functional losses, often assessed in glaucoma with visual field examination. Both structural and functional changes result from a common pathophysiological process, namely loss of retinal ganglion cells (RGC) and their axons.[4] Structure-function relationships are central to what clinicians do day in and day out managing glaucoma patients. At a basic level, such correlations have enabled us to better understand the course of glaucoma and its pathogenesis. As more sophisticated diagnostic techniques have emerged, correlating the structural findings with the outcomes of functional tests such as perimetry have made it possible to diagnose glaucoma sooner or detect signs of glaucoma with more confidence. Much has been discussed in the glaucoma literature about whether signs of structural damage precede functional evidence of glaucomatous injury to retinal ganglion cells. Early publications suggested that there is a significant amount of redundancy with regard to the RGC in the human eye and therefore up to 40% of retinal ganglion cells could be lost before signs of damage are observed on standard achromatic perimetry,[5] a technique that remains the current gold standard for detection of functional loss in glaucoma patients.

An important histological study on which this observation was based included a very small number of eyes.[5] It is a common clinical observation that signs of structural damage at the level of the optic nerve head (ONH), RNFL, or macula can be established before definitive signs of visual field loss are observed on standard automated perimetry (SAP).[6,7] The reverse is also occasionally true, i.e., signs of VF loss can manifest before definitive signs of damage can be observed in glaucoma. For example in the European Glaucoma Prevention Study, more eyes developed VF loss as the earliest sign of glaucoma.[8] However, it is possible that some of these eyes from EGPS already had structural glaucomatous damage not detected by the subjective assessment of disc stereo-photographs. The structure and function relationship seems to be mostly nonlinear especially in early glaucoma where minimal signs of functional damage, as assessed by SAP, are expected to be present before a sizable proportion of the RGCs have already been lost.

Based on many recent studies, it is now understood that the apparent non-linear relationship seen between structural and functional signs of glaucoma is probably a manifestation of the different scaling units of structural and functional tests as well as the different variability of the two types of measures. For example, while perimetric assessment is usually performed with logarithmic units, structural parameters are usually given in linear units. When perimetric sensitivities are averaged in linear units the relation with rim area becomes more linear.[9] While no significant relationship has been reported between structural and functional outcomes in normal subjects, when the visual field sensitivity is expressed in linear units (1/L) instead of dB units, a direct linear relationship has been seen in both experimental glaucoma in monkeys[10] and humans.[9] Below we will discuss various models that have been suggested for describing structure function relationships in glaucoma.

3.1.2. Current proposed models linking structure and function in glaucoma

3.1.2.1. Harwerth *et al.*'s model: VF threshold sensitivity vs. RGC density

Studies by Harwerth *et al.*[1] have uniquely contributed to our understanding of SF relationships by correlating histological RGC counts with visual field sensitivities (expressed in linear 1/L units) both derived from experimental glaucoma induced in monkeys.[1] The investigators demonstrated a linear relationship between the

RGC count and visual field sensitivity in the central retina. Interestingly, the slope of this correlation increased as a function of eccentricity. The latter finding is likely a function of the changing distribution of the RGCs in the central macula. This points to a proportional relationship between the two measures with a certain percentage of RGC loss corresponding to a similar percentage of VF sensitivity loss. This is consistent with the two-stage mode as introduced by Swanson *et al.*[11] The latter posits that if both RGC loss and perimetric sensitivities are expressed in percent loss, the relationship will be linear at least for spatial filters in the range of 0.5-2 cycles/degrees are involved; however the slope of the linear relationship varies as a function of distance from fixation. This finding may be one of the explanations for the bipartite model as described by Drasdo and colleagues.[12] Alternatively, the relationship between size of the Goldmann III stimulus with Ricco's critical area could explain this change in slope. The critical area is the size of the area within the retina where spatial summation is complete. Ricco's area is smaller than the stimulus size III area more centrally, where as it becomes larger as more and more peripheral locations are tested. For stimulus areas larger than the critical area (such as stimulus size III centrally), sensitivity changes less and therefore, the slope for the correlation of RGC density or thickness and VF sensitivity is shallower. Pan and Swanson have recently suggested that detection of the target by multiple cortical spatial filters could explain this relationship as well.[13]

3.1.2.2. The Hood-Kardon model (simple linear model)

The Hood-Kardon model essentially is based on the premise that structural measures, most notably RNFL, consist of a neural component, mostly RGC axons, and a non-neural component consisting of glial tissues, blood vessels and other connective tissue elements. As glaucoma advances, the neural component of the RNFL thins out while the non-neural component remains stable and could actually increase in thickness. This assumption had also been previously modeled by Harwerth *et al.*[1] It defines a dynamic range for the SF relationship where the relationship between structural and functional measures is linear, when visual field data is expressed on a linear scale, a finding similar to those of Harwerth *et al.*[1] In this model, structural measures asymptotically tend towards their floor of measurements around when about 90% of the visual function has originally been lost (*i.e.*, around -10 dB); from this point on, the structural measures are so thin and there is significant noise in the segmentation that monitoring structural measures such as RNFL would become very difficult.

3.1.2.3. The 'Hockey-Stick' model: changing slope of SF relationship as a function of eccentricity

This model takes into account that the relationship between sensitivity and ganglion cell receptive fields density is linear, but varies according to eccentricity (slope of 1 at greater eccentricities and a slope of 0.16 in the macula). Overall, a two-line or 'Hockey-Stick' fit gives a reasonable fit to the data, and it resembles the spatial summation curves which predicted a shallower slope for test locations near fixation and a steeper slope peripherally. The change in slope may be explained by the relationship between the size of Goldmann III stimulus in relation to the critical area (Ricco's area). For stimulus area larger than Ricco's area, which is the case in the central 15 degrees, sensitivity changes less. Although probability summation of neural detectors is the most accepted explanation, the detection of the stimulus by multiple cortical spatial filters may also be considered as an alternative explanation.[4]

Drasdo *et al.*'s model:[3] The bipartite model linking RGC density to VF sensitivity also addresses the displacement of the RGCs within the central macula as pertains correspondence with the central VF test locations. Drasdo and colleagues used histological data on lateral displacement of RCG bodies from foveal cones to develop an improved map of normal ganglion cell density within the central visual field. They proposed a model relating ganglion cell receptive fields densities to perimetric sensitivities. This model has linear contrast sensitivity linearly related to ganglion cell densities for perimetric values of 0 to 29 dB, then becomes non-linear at higher sensitivities. This nonlinear part of the model predicts a shallower structure-function slope in the macula area, and an increase in slope in the peripheral retina.

3.1.3. Factors affecting the structure-function relationships

As both structural and functional changes result from a common pathophysiological process (loss of RGC somas and axons), it would be expected that both would be related to one another over the course of disease. However, the current structural and functional measurement methods show considerable variability, acquire measurements in different scales, and are susceptible to limitations that result in a suboptimal assessment of this relationship, which is dependent on the severity of the disease and the location being tested.

Automated imaging devices are often used for structural assessment (ONH, RNFL, macula), aiming to quantify rim area (mm^2), RNFL thickness (microns), or various inner retinal thickness measures (microns). These represent linear metrics of measurements, and should be linearly related to RGC density. Standard automated perimetry (SAP) uses a constant size stimulus at all test locations, and VF sensitivity is obtained in logarithmic units (decibels – dB). The dB is relative to a reference level (luminance of the stimulus vs. background luminance), and it is used to express a ratio rather than an absolute value. Thus, dB is a non-linear measure, and a change of 3 dB represents a doubling or halving of light intensity. When dB increments are plotted against a linear scale, it shows that dB increments at different levels of intensity represent very different sized increments on a linear scale. For example, a 2-dB decrease from 38 to 36 dB is ten-fold greater change in linear units than the same dB change at a sensitivity of 28 dB. The different units of measurements for structural and functional parameters are confounding factors when assessing structure-function relationship. There is strong evidence based on experimental and clinical studies that transforming dB to linear scale results in a clearer linear relationship between structure and function measurements. Nevertheless, it is important to understand that the logarithmic scale compresses the range of losses in early stages, while expanding the range in later stages. Although a linearization of the visual field data suggests that functional changes may occur at early stages of disease process, the simple linearization may not yield improvement in the detection of early functional losses because SAP data is originally acquired using staircase procedures based on logarithmic scale (decibels).[14] Thus, current implementations of SAP are not effective in detecting small amounts of RGC loss in early stages of disease. On the other hand, by expanding the range of the scale at later stages, SAP may be more sensitive to small RGC loss that do not seem to produce detectable changes in RNFL thickness.[15]

Visual field measurements show significant between-subject variability. Perimetric indices have normal ranges that cover a substantial portion of linear scale. In addition, visual field assessment is a psychophysical evaluation that shows considerable test-retest variability. For perimetry with size III, test-retest variability of perimetric sensitivity in *damaged* areas of the visual field can span the entire dynamic range of the perimeter. These combined sources of variability affecting functional measurements confound structure-function relationship, particularly in the assessment of glaucomatous change over time. The determination of visual field sensitivity is dependent on the stimulus area (spatial summation), as when small areas of retina are stimulated, the area of the retina stimulated is linearly related to the visual sensitivity (Ricco's law). One caveat is that this small area (Ricco's area) varies according to the location of the retina being stimulated (eccentricity), whereas within 15° from fixation this area is smaller than the Goldmann size III stimulus used on SAP. In addition, cortical pooling of ganglion cell responses can be characterized in terms of multiple spatial mechanisms or multiple cortical detectors with peak responses at different spatial frequency. A decline in ganglion cells density reduces the sensitivity of higher frequency cortical spatial mechanism mediating detection in normal eyes. Cortical pooling analysis demonstrates that this reduction in sensitivity of higher frequency mechanisms would result in a linear decline in sensitivity with decline in ganglion cell density. Thus, the sensitivity to the size III stimulus may decline with modest amount of ganglion cell loss, with a shallower slope in the central visual field when compared to a steeper slope at the periphery.[11]

Another confounding source is the concept of 'ganglion cell dysfunction' (rather than death). In some situations, RGC may become dysfunctional leading to a functional deficit response at that time, which may or may not be reversible. In this situation, measured functional abnormalities may exceed functional impairment predicted from structural measurement alone. Electrophysiological studies showed that a reversible reduction of PERG amplitude could be induced by elevating intraocular pressure[16] and that IOP reduction can result in functional improvement. Psychophysical evidence of RGC dysfunction is consistent with shrinkage of dendritic fields.[17] Structural measurements lso show significant between-subject variability. Ganglion cell number in normal human eyes varies by a factor of two across individuals, and structural indices have considerably wide normal ranges.[11] Although test-retest variability is low, it can further enlarge the between-subject variability. The test-retest variability may be due to operator, instrument, or patient-related causes, and some locations may show wider measurement variability in some imaging modalities (*i.e.*, OCT RNFL at temporal and nasal quadrants). The variability in structural (and functional) measurements makes the true extent of damage difficult to ascertain, which represent a relevant confounding source for the assessment of structure-function relationship over time.

Although imaging measurements of neuroretinal rim and RNFL thickness are related to RGC loss, these structural measurements include non-neural elements such as glial tissue and blood vessels. In eyes in which visual function drops to zero, anatomical measures have a residual non-neural component that can be considered substantial even in blind eyes (35-55 microns for peripapillary RNFL).[18,19] There are uncertainties concerning the extent of the non-neural components of the RNFL, and how these may be affected by age and disease severity. Axon diameter and density vary around the optic nerve head circumference, which implies that the number of axons according to RNFL thickness varies around the ONH circumference, and this relationship may be affected by age. The residual non-neural component seems to be smaller in the neuroretinal rim than RNFL, but the morphology of ONH varies considerably between individuals and rim measurements may be affected by biomechanical changes of peripapillary sclera and lamina cribrosa.

The spatial structure-function relationship requires knowledge about the anatomical correspondence of neuroretinal rim, or peripapillary RNFL, to the visual field test locations. Garway-Heath *et al.* proposed one of the most utilized structure-function maps.[9] These authors and others have observed that the position of the ONH relative to the fovea, disc size, and axial length were the most important factors influencing the trajectory of RNFL bundles.[20] Also, there appears to be a considerable variability around the ONH entry point for a given VF location, spanning 20-30 degrees.[21] Moreover, the location of the temporal raphe may also vary among individuals, considerably affecting the spatial structure-function correspondence. In fact, these various sources of between-subject variability likely represent a major cause of imprecision in the evaluation of spatial structure-function relationship. Adaptation of the spatial correspondence map to include factors that help explain individual variation in the correspondence of retinal locations to peripapillary RNFL sectors and temporal raphe location would further improve spatial structure-function associations.[4]

3.1.4. Future directions

Combining structure-function testing improves the diagnostic ability to detect glaucoma and glaucoma progression. Structure and function measurement methods have several confounding factors that preclude a better integration of both tests results. Attempts to improve the assessment of this complex relationship would include improvements of structural tests technology, adaptations of visual field tests, and better approaches for combining the information provided by both tests.

Ideally, rapidly evolving imaging technology may allow a quantitative assessment of RCG nuclei *in vivo*, permitting direct comparison with retinal sensitivity. Visual field test points in conventional 24-2 grid could then be modified to better represent the distribution of RGCs, and also, the stimulus size could be 'scaled' by estimates of RGC receptive field density across the central 30 degrees.

Meanwhile, Medeiros *et al.*[15,22] recently proposed a new method to estimate rates of RGC loss in glaucoma by combining structural and functional measurements. Estimates of RGC count were obtained from functional and structural tests data (SAP and OCT, respectively). RGC count estimated from SAP data accounted for eccentricity of each tested point, and considered cell density to be uniform over an area of retina corresponding to an area of 6 x 6 degrees of visual field space that separates test locations in SAP. RGC count estimated from OCT data accounted for the effect of aging in the axonal density and the effect of disease severity on the relationship between the neuronal and non-neuronal components of the RNFL thickness as obtained by OCT. Then, a weighted average of both RGC estimates were obtained based on the severity of disease (as assessed by MD values), whereas in early disease, OCT-derived RGC estimates have greater weight than those obtained by SAP; and in advanced disease, SAP estimates will carry greater weight than those obtained from OCT. The age-related loss of estimated RGC loss was calculated from data obtained in 52 healthy eyes followed-up longitudinally for 4.0 (± 0.7) years. The authors of this study observed that the rate of RGC loss estimated by this model performed better than either isolated structural or functional measures for detecting progressive glaucomatous change.

3.2. Structure and function topographical maps: Which one should we rely on?

3.2.1. Introduction

Both structural and functional assessments are used widely for the diagnosis and management of glaucoma. The most commonly used functional assessment is visual field testing, which typically estimates sensitivity to visual stimuli (most commonly small circular luminance increments) that are sampled at a series of locations across the central approximately 30 degrees of visual field. Structural assessments are varied, but typically include assessment of the optic nerve head via photography or optical coherence tomography (OCT), OCT measurement of retinal nerve fiber layer thickness measurement in the peripapillary area, and OCT assessment of the thickness of various retinal layers in the macular region. In order to compare the outcomes of functional assessments to structural assessments, a mapping schema between the two is required. Here we discuss current mapping schema that are used for the purpose of enabling registration between functional and structural assays. We will discuss the two mapping challenges that are currently most important for glaucoma: (1) mapping from points in visual field space to the likely angle of insertion of the relevant RGC axons on the optic nerve head; and (2) mapping from points in visual field space to retinal ganglion cell complex thickness in the macular region. Other sections will discuss how to combine measures of structure and function.

3.2.2. Mapping between visual field space and the relevant sector on the optic nerve head

3.2.2.1. The methods used to derive maps

Several approaches have been used to derive maps between visual field space and the optic nerve head. The most commonly used methods have been: (1) visual inspection/tracing of retinal nerve fiber bundles (or the absence of RNFL bundles in eyes with glaucoma) related to overlaid maps of visual field test locations (for example: see refs. 9, 21 and 23) (2) computational models incorporating knowledge of ocular;[23,24] (3) statistical approaches investigating the strength of correlations between locations in visual field space and anatomical damage at the ONH;[25,26] and (4) combinations of the above.[27,28] The results of all these modelling approaches yield similar results for the 'average' eye. Each approach has limitations. For example, visual inspection of photographs is limited by image quality and has been shown to have limited reproducabillity even when conducted by experienced clinicians[29] and computational modelling requires the incorporation of a range of assumptions that may not hold for individual eyes. Nevertheless, there is relatively strong agreement in the mapping produced by all approaches as would be expected by the reasonably consistent basic features of ocular anatomy.

3.2.2.2. 'One size fits all' versus 'one size fits one'

The usage of such structure function maps within clinical instrumentation and analysis currently uses a 'one size fits all' approach, where the map provided is for the 'average person'. A commonly-used approach incorporates the map of Garway-Heath *et al.*[9] (2000) that maps the 24-2 visual field to six sectors on the optic disc. Such mapping schema provide useful estimates of an approximate area

within the research domain with substantial additional empirical work required to ascertain whether there is indeed clinical utility in such an approach.

3.3. Detecting glaucoma by structural versus functional tests. Does structural damage precede detectable functional loss? What is the evidence?

3.3.1. Statement of aim

Clinicians generally believe that structural damage precedes functional defects in glaucoma. The goal of this section is to review the basis and evidence for this belief.

Estimates of the accuracy of structural or functional tests to detect glaucoma depend on the reference standard used.[43,44] Unfortunately, there is no single gold standard reference test for the detection of glaucoma. Studies evaluating the structural tests use functional tests as the reference standard while the studies evaluating functional tests use structural assessment as the reference standard. It is therefore difficult to compare the ability of structural and functional tests to detect glaucoma directly. An indirect way of comparing the ability of structural and functional tests to detect glaucoma is to compare the sensitivity and specificity of the criterion used to define glaucoma in the published literature. Sample *et al.* evaluated the sensitivity of various vision function tests to identify glaucoma (using progressive glaucomatous optic neuropathy on serial photographs as the reference standard) and found them to have a sensitivity of 50-65% at a specificity level of 80%.[45] The sensitivity levels were much lower at a specificity level of 90%. This meant that 35-50% of subjects with glaucomatous optic neuropathy (as detected by subjective optic disc photographic assessment) had no detectable vision function loss. Most of the studies evaluating the diagnostic ability of structural tests (imaging methods, spectral domain OCT being the most popular method currently) have used visual fields and the presence of glaucomatous optic neuropathy as the reference standard for glaucoma. Studies evaluating the diagnostic ability of SD-OCT (using visual fields alone as the reference standard) have reported sensitivities between 60-80% at a specificity level of 80%.[46-48] This meant that 20-40% of subjects with repeatable perimetric defects had no detectable structural abnormality on SD-OCT.

It is often believed that structural changes occur before functional changes in glaucoma, based on the work by Quigley *et al.*[5,49] and Sommer *et al.*[50] A recent study supported this by showing that eyes eventually developing glaucomatous VF defect had significantly lower RNFL thickness compared to healthy eyes up to eight years before the development of glaucomatous VF defect.[51] However, multiple studies have demonstrated contradicting results. Malik *et al.* analyzed the data from the studies by Quigley *et al.* and showed that many eyes with normal retinal ganglion cell (RGC) counts had abnormal mean deviation (MD) on automated perimetry.[46] Three eyes had RGC counts greater than 100% with MD worse than -5 dB. Large clinical trials in eyes with ocular hypertension and early glaucoma have shown that functional changes can precede optic nerve head changes in a significant number of patients.[8,52,53] It should be noted, however, that it is possible that structural assessment was based on subjective evaluation of disc photos. It is possible that many of these eyes already had structural damage at baseline. Histological data from monkey eyes also has shown that perimetric defects can be present in very early stages of glaucoma, and a sensitivity loss of greater than 5 dB can be present for minimal amounts of ganglion cell loss.[10] Whether structural or functional change occurs first also depends on the chosen endpoints and how they are measured. Also some disagreement might be always expected due to the asynchronous temporal relationship between retinal ganglion cell functional and structural decline in the glaucomatous process.[54] The concept of 'ganglion cell dysfunction' (rather than death) has been proposed to explain why, in some patients, perimetric defects precede identifiable structural changes. In early stages of ganglion cell insult, cells may become dysfunctional, leading to a reduction in visual field sensitivity, so that 'measured structure' may not be representative of functioning ganglion cell or axonal number.[4]

In spite of the above equivocal evidence, there is no contradicting the fact that retinal nerve fiber layer abnormalities (either on photographs or on imaging methods) are present in many cases with normal visual fields. The reasons for this finding are elaborately explained in a few previous reports.[2,4,14,55] In clinical practice, when we are interested in finding out which test will show statistically significant glaucomatous damage first, then the answer depends upon the relative variability in the test measurements of structure and function among normal eyes. A test with a larger standard deviation among normal eyes, all else being equal, would require a larger change to reach statistical significance than would a test with a smaller standard deviation. It has been debated whether much of the apparently earlier change in structure derives from greater variability in field test data.

3.4. How should clinicians follow glaucoma suspects over time with structural and functional tests?

3.4.1. Statement of aim

This summary aims to discuss general guidelines on how to monitor patients with suspected glaucoma using current commercially available technologies. The present summary will not address the sensitivity and specificity of structural vs. functional tests, which is the topic of another summary discussion within this section. For the same reason, the issue of disagreement between technologies will not be discussed here. The underlying assumption of this summary is that glaucoma is best diagnosed based upon conclusive abnormalities seen on functional AND/OR structural tests.

Patients are often deemed 'glaucoma suspects' when structural or functional tests do not provide conclusive information regarding the presence (or absence) of glaucomatous (or 'glaucoma-like') abnormalities. Some clinicians and researchers advocate that patients can be deemed suspects either due to suspicious optic discs (based either on appearance and/or imaging), visual fields falling in the gray zone of being neither normal nor abnormal, or elevated intraocular pressure (ocular hypertension). This summary will include this broader definition of glaucoma suspects and the statements proposed herewith may be applicable to both cases. Moreover, glaucoma suspects can be further stratified based on their risk of glaucoma onset. For ocular hypertensives, objective risk models are available to estimate their five-year risk of conversion to primary open-angle glaucoma. Such feature is not yet available for suspects based on disc appearance. Nonetheless, clinicians can stratify these patients based on known risk factors for glaucoma development and progression, such as race, family history, age, central corneal thickness, and findings from objective imaging technologies.

Since glaucoma is by definition a progressive disease, following-up glaucoma suspects over time with structural and functional tests will provide conclusive information about the presence (or absence, so far) of glaucomatous damage. In addition, all structural and functional diagnostic tests have inherent limitations, one of which is their imperfect repeatability, even when reliability and quality indices are adequate. For instance, a patient may be deemed a 'suspect' based upon a given test result during a baseline assessment. Upon repeated testing some weeks later, the repeat test on the same modality may now demonstrate more conclusive signs of glaucomatous damage not attributed to progression, but rather to variability (or learning effect) known to exist for that modality.

A recipe for following glaucoma suspects should provide guidance on: which clinical and auxiliary tests should be performed, at what intervals, should these intervals be kept constant in years to come, should follow-up continue indefinitely in those who have not converted (yet?).

Therefore, the answer to 'how clinicians should follow glaucoma suspects over time with structural and functional tests' depends upon two main factors: (1) the speed (rate of change) of deterioration; (2) the test-retest variability of the technologies available in their clinical setting; and (3) their estimated risk of glaucoma development, whether based on objective or subjective methods as described above.

In consonance with the 8th consensus of the WGA on glaucoma progression, "corroboration of glaucomatous progression [or onset] through the use of more than one test may provide more effective and more rapid detection of glaucomatous progression [or onset] than repeated confirmation of change using a single modality." This statement addresses the first part of the question this summary aims to discuss. Note that, although we introduced the term 'onset' to the original WGA statement, that same document supports that conversion from normality to glaucoma also involves progressive changes due to the same underlying mechanism, that is, death of retinal ganglion cells (RGC).

For simplicity, we herewith assume that static perimetry (*i.e.*, standard automated perimetry, SAP) is the most widely available and accepted functional test, whereas optic disc photography (with or without adjunctive imaging technologies) is the structural counterpart. Since patients with ocular hypertension have normal SAP and disc photography results, which minimizes classification bias that would come from using either test to define a suspect, follow-up of these patients provide valuable insight on the frequency SAP and disc photography can detect early glaucomatous damage. In the Ocular Hypertension Treatment Study (OHTS), a similar number of participants were classified as having converted to primary open-angle glaucoma based on disc photos and SAP. Therefore, our second statement adds to the first one that, SAP and disc photography should be repeated over time in patients with suspected glaucoma.

Although frequency doubling technology (FDT) has been shown useful to diagnose glaucoma, there is currently no data suggesting that it can replace SAP or even that it should be performed alongside SAP when both techniques are available. The same principles can be applied to electrophysiological tests, such as multifocal visual evoked potentials (mfVEP) and pattern electroretinogram for glaucoma (PERGLA). Despite their more objective assessment of visual function and ability to detect damage sometimes before SAP, these tests can be used when following glaucoma suspects as an adjunct to SAP as a means to provide a function-function corroboration (also in consonance with the 8th consensus statement above). If available, these adjunctive functional tests could be alternated with SAP during follow up of glaucoma suspects.

Optical coherence tomography (OCT), is currently the most widely employed, commercially-available adjunctive structural test to monitor suspects over time. Its performance to detect glaucoma, as well as other adjunctive structural technologies, is discussed elsewhere in this section. Some patients may reveal significant structural abnormalities consistent with glaucoma before functional defects. The objective nature of OCT may also reveal abnormalities overlooked on optic disc photography. Similarly to the discussion above on functional tests, if available, OCT could be alternated with optic disc photography during follow up of glaucoma suspects.

3.4.2. Frequency of testing

The test-retest variability of the techniques described above should be considered when defining how frequently they should be performed over time in glaucoma suspects. One should keep in mind that this variability has an inherent component but also depends on patient-related factors. Some patient-related components include: disease severity, clarity of media, and cooperativeness during the test. As far as severity, glaucoma suspects by definition have normal or almost-normal test results and thus are assumed to have lower short- as well as long-term variability. For the remaining components, we will assume optimal for simplification purposes.

Assuming that at least two baseline tests with acceptable reliability indices were initially performed, the frequency of repeated testing will depend upon the disease progression and the test variability, as discussed above. The recommendations by Chauhan *et al.*[56] on measuring rates of visual field change in glaucoma provide some insight that can be extrapolated (with caution) when monitoring visual field changes in glaucoma suspects. Assuming a low degree of variability in this population, a frequency of two 24-2 SAP examinations per year would allow the detection of moderately to rapidly deteriorating visual field MD (-0.5 to -2.0 dB/yr) in up to five years of follow-up with a power of 80%. For slowly deteriorating fields (-0.25 dB/yr), the same can be achieved in 6.5 years. Although these recommendations are based on averaged pooled data, we believe they provide a robust estimate for the purpose of this summary. These recommendations are also based on a global visual field index (MD), which despite not providing focal information, has the advantage of being less variable over time. Recommendations based on focal changes are not yet available and would need to take into account its inherent larger variability – although a much larger number of VF locations could be analyzed. For the moment, we propose that performing two visual field examinations per year should not have an onerous impact on patients (nor insurer) and could provide a high degree of certainty to detect conversion from suspected to glaucomatous visual fields among high-risk patients during the course of a five-year follow-up period.

Regarding disc photography, one key limitation is its subjective nature between and within graders over time. There are currently no studies addressing the optimal frequency of testing to detect conversion from a normal/suspicious disc to a conclusively abnormal one. Aside from the increased chances of detecting disc hemorrhages upon very frequent photography, structural changes detectable by the human eye are often subtle and very slow in glaucoma. A recommendation on the frequency of disc photographs in glaucoma suspects should therefore take into account the balance between how onerous it is to patients and how long it would take to identify minimally-detectable changes. One alternative is to try and extrapolate this choice on the frequency of visual field test, for which more data exist. By performing one disc photograph per year, clinicians should be able to confront their impression while looking at two disc photographs with a sequence of at least two repeatable (or confirmatory) visual field examinations.

OCT has a number of advantages over disc photography and visual field testing, namely its more objective nature and lower test-retest variability. These features give them a theoretical advantage to detect conversion from normal/suspects to glaucoma. They can help not only by providing structure-function corroboration, but also structure-structure corroboration with optic photographs. With a smaller test-retest variability and the possibility to confront with other functional and structural tests, ancillary structural tests could be performed once a year, possibly six months after disc photography and concomitant to one of the visual field tests.

Although in clinical practice clinicians have become increasingly more dependent on OCT compared the disc photographs for diagnosis and monitoring of glaucoma, the latter still provides fundamental information in a clinical setting. One important issue is disc hemorrhage detection, as OCT cannot detect it yet. Another issue are the nerve fiber layer defects seen on photographs which can be compared with OCT results to detect abnormality or detect progression. Further, we may miss retinal abnormalities or other optic neuropathies which may mimic glaucomatous changes if optic disc photographies are not performed.

3.5. Changes in perimetry to incorporate structural information

3.5.1. Statement of aim

While both functional and structural information are considered to diagnose glaucoma, perimetric and imaging methods have largely been developed independently of each other. There may, however, be a benefit to using structural information to inform visual field testing. The goal of this section is to review perimetric approaches that incorporate structural information.

3.5.1.1. Advantages of presenting structural and functional information together

Hood *et al.*[57] developed a customized one-page report containing key features of optical coherent tomography (OCT) scans and visual field information. They suggest that an advantage of such report includes the ease of looking for topographical consistency between structural and functional parameters. Furthermore, the direct comparison of the topography of visual field and OCT abnormalities may lead to the detection of subtle damage that may otherwise be ignored. Structure-function reports that include information from the OCT macular cube scans can lead to the detection of glaucomatous damage to the macula. Including a large scan image on the report allows for the detection of algorithm errors and structural abnormalities. Hood *et al.*[57] showed excellent inter-individual repeatability between two report specialists (individuals experienced in analyzing OCT and VF results) and also excellent diagnostic ability compared to glaucoma specialists.

Presenting RNFL thickness plot in the NSTIN format instead of the TSNIT format. Hood *et al.*[57] suggested that presenting RNFL information in the NSTIN format makes it easier to relate thinning on the RNFL plot to central defects on the visual field.

Commercially available perimetric outputs that include structural information. Combined structural and functional information are included on some commercially available devices. The advantages of this include increased availability of structure-function reports to a large number of clinicians and the usefulness of the reports for patient education.

The Polar Analysis. This analysis is available on the OCTOPUS perimeters (Haag-Streit, Switzerland) and provides a graphical representation of the relationship between structural and functional results. The pattern of locations tested using the G test was selected based on the anatomical distribution of the retinal nerve fiber layer bundle. The Polar Analysis plots the visual field results obtained at each location in their corresponding location along the optic disc. The length of the bars represents the magnitude of the defect. Green bars represent visual field locations that have significantly better results while red bars represent visual field locations that have significantly worse results than age-matched controls. This graphical representation allows clinicians to quickly assess the correspondence between the visual field results and structure.

Cluster Analysis. This analysis is available on the OCTOPUS perimeters (Haag-Streit, Switzerland) and provides a graphical representation of the relationship between structural and functional results. In the Cluster Analysis, visual field locations corresponding to the same retinal nerve fiber layer (RNFL) bundle are averaged to provide a mean defect for each of ten clusters.

The Heidelberg Edge Perimeter (HEP). This perimeter performs standards automated perimetry and also flicker-defined form perimetry. The HEYEX software allows the integration of the visual field results with optic nerve head and RNFL information obtained with the Heidelberg HRT and Spectralis devices. This integration allows for a combined analysis of structural and functional status, with all information presented on a single report generated by the HEYEX software.

3.5.1.2. Fundus-guided perimetry (often referred to as microperimetry) may be useful for glaucoma diagnosis, but requires an adequate understanding of the structure-function mapping

Fundus-guided perimetry allows for an assessment of visual function under direct observation of the fundus. With this type of perimetry, visual function can be tested at specific structural loci with possibly reduced test-retest variability in the positioning of the stimulus on the retina. Fundus-guided perimetry has been shown to be useful in the assessment of visual function in macular diseases and is of value as a functional outcome measure in clinical trials of geographic atrophy. Fundus-guided perimetry may have role in glaucoma but it requires an adequate understanding of structure-function mapping in order to accurately predict areas of interest to test. An important difference between macular diseases and glaucoma is the degree of spatial congruence between the affected area of the retina and the associated location of dysfunction in visual function. Whereas there is high congruence in retinal diseases, this is not the case for glaucoma. Nevertheless, the fixation tracking technology associated with fundus-guided perimetry may prove useful for perimetric testing in glaucoma to minimize the effects of small eye movements on test-retest variability, even if the specific locations of the stimulus presentation are not chosen on an individualized basis (*i.e.*, the test is not truly 'fundus-guided').

Currently, fundus-guided perimetry can be performed using the following commercially available devices: the Nidek Microperimeters58 (Nidek Technologies Srl., Padua, Italy), Macular Integrity Assessment (MAIA)59 (CenterVue, Padova, Italy), and Compass[60] (CenterVue, Padova, Italy).

Increasing the number of test points in areas where structural defects are present may be useful to diagnose glaucoma. There is a trade-off between the time needed to perform a perimetric test and the number of locations that can be assessed. This places a limit on the spatial resolution of perimetry, or in other words, the number of visual field locations that can be assessed. Some evidence suggests that it may be useful to identify areas of the visual field that should be tested with a more densely packed grid based on structural information.

Increasing the number of test points in the macula may be useful to diagnose glaucoma. Hood *et al.* have shown the presence of visual loss in the macula in patients with glaucoma.[61] They showed that if retinal ganglion cell displacement is accounted for, a direct comparison between retinal nerve fiber layer and visual field defects is possible. These macular defects in visual function were identified using the 10-2 test. While performing the 10-2 in addition to the 24-2 test may provide useful diagnostic information, this is not practical from a clinical standpoint. Ehrlich *et al.* therefore modified the 24-2 test to include some points from the 10-2.[62] They noted the following advantages to modifying the 24-2 test instead of developing a new test: (1) a 24-2 report could be generated to allow longitudinal;

follow-up; (2) the 10-2 normative data is already collected and could be used; (3) the results of the additional 10-2 locations in the modified test pattern could be compared directly to the same locations in the 10-2 test. Higher sensitivity at a fixed specificity of 85% was observed even when only four addition 10-2 points were added to the 24-2 test pattern.[62] Chen *et al.* also showed that testing two additional locations in the superior macula can improve the detection of glaucoma using the test pattern available on the Medmont perimeter.[63]

On the Octopus perimeter, the pattern used in the G test has a larger number of central points compared to the HFA 24-2 test. The pattern of the G test is based on the retinal nerve fiber bundles and contains has a higher density of point in the central area to detect foveal and para-central defects.

Using structural information to identify regions to test with a dense test grid. In different patients, glaucoma is first detected by either the presence of structural abnormalities, the presence of functional loss, or by both simultaneously.[8,64] In patients where a structural abnormality is detected before functional loss, it may be valuable to monitor the area of the visual field that corresponds to the area of structural defect. Customized tests could be used to test a smaller area of the visual field with a denser grid. This could result in the detection of very early visual loss. While no normative data would be available for such tests, patients could serve as their own baseline in longitudinal follow-up. Algorithms, such as the experimental scotoma-oriented perimetry (SCOPE)[65] or the gradient-oriented automated natural neighbor approach (GOANNA)[66] could be developed and automated provide a higher density assessment of relevant visual field areas.

Research on improving perimetry using structural information may lead to clinical perimetric methods that will improve glaucoma diagnosis in the future. There are a number of approaches that have been, and continue to be, explored in the academic setting. These approaches, while promising, currently have a fairly limited evidence base and are not currently ready for implementation in clinical settings. Some of these approaches are described below.

Biasing the prior of a Bayesian test procedure based on structure. Denniss *et al.*[67] have explored the ability of using patient-specific prior information such as structural damage to improve perimetric procedures. In the structure-zippy estimation by sequential testing (SZEST), they biased the prior of a Bayesian procedure with information from structural imaging using computer simulations.

3.6.3. *Appraisal of current methods*

Several approaches have been proposed to combine results from structural and functional tests to improve detection of glaucoma and glaucoma progression.

3.6.3.1. Method #1: Bayesian methods

Bayesian statistics provide an objective, quantitative method that allows different sources of information to be pooled.[74] They are based on the concept that prior information can be used to modify posterior beliefs using a formula known as Baye's theorem.[75] Using Bayesian statistics, information obtained from one type of test (*e.g.*, OCT) can provide a prior probability of disease (or of disease progression) that can be used to influence conclusions obtained from another test (*e.g.*, SAP). For example, a change in visual field that may be deemed statistically insignificant on its own may be considered significant after taking into account structural changes in the same eye. The method can also be applied to rates of change over time. Several investigators have explored combining information from structural and functional tests in glaucoma using Bayesian methods.[74,76,77]

Medeiros *et al.* used a Bayesian model to classify eyes as progressing or non-progressing using combined information from SAP and average RNFL thickness measurements from scanning laser polarimetry (SLP).[77] The combined approach identified a greater number of eyes as progressing compared to ordinary least squares regression methods used by software of commercially available visual field and OCT devices. Sensitivity of the method to detect progression was also tested in a group of eyes classified as progressing on optic disc stereo-photographs, achieving a sensitivity of 74% compared to only 37% using the ordinary least squares regression. The Bayesian method had excellent specificity, correctly identify 100% of 29 healthy eyes as not progressing. In a subsequent work, Russell *et al.* found that measurements of neuroretinal rim area from CSLO could be used to improve the estimate of rate of change in visual field over time in patients with ocular hypertension.[74] The rate of change in rim area was calculated using linear regression and the slope of change used as a 'prior' to inform the rate of change in SAP mean sensitivity using Bayesian linear regression. The Bayesian method was better able to predict future change in SAP compared to the trend analysis of SAP measurements alone. However, a limitation of this method is that the differences in measurement scales between CSLO and SAP needed to be overcome by transforming the CSLO data using a scaling factor derived from the same patient sample, introducing a possible source of error.[74] Medeiros *et al.* also used a Bayesian joint regression model to combine information from CSLO and SAP in patients with glaucoma. The Bayesian slopes of change over time were more accurate predictors of future visual field than conventional ordinary least squares regression of the isolated measures.[76]

Advantages

Advantages of Bayesian methods are that they provide a means for correlation between tests to be formally taken into account. This can help deal with conflicting results and provide confirmation of change when results are in agreement. On the other hand they also reduce the chances of a type-1 error, *i.e.*, the probability of declaring a change significant that has actually occurred by chance. Bayesian methods also reduce the problems of the variability inherent in all testing modalities. Variability increases the number of tests needed to accurately identify change. For example, some eyes with relatively fast rates of visual field loss may be declared non-progressing by conventional ordinary least squares regression due to variability of the test. In statistical terms this would be evident from the large standard error of the regression slope. In such circumstances, more measurements would be needed to accurately determine the rate of change, which would result in increased time and financial costs for the clinician and patient and potentially delay recognition of true change. By combining information from different tests it is possible to reduce the effect of variability in the individual tests. Bayesian methods also allow information regarding risk factors such as IOP and CCT to be incorporated.[15]

Limitations

A limitation of Bayesian methods is that they do not overcome all of the difficulties of different measurement scales of structural and functional tests. When used to examine rates of change over time, methods described to date, also assume a linear rate of change in both domains. Functional changes are probably not linear given the logarithmic scale of SAP and the effects of spatial summation in the retina.[4,78]

3.6.3.2. Method #2: Transforming structural and function measurements to find a common domain

Several approaches have been described that attempt to overcome the difficulties of measurement scale when combining information from structural and functional tests and express results in the same domain.[22,69,74] For example, Zhu *et al.* developed a method of predicting visual field sensitivity from structural measurements using a type of neural network.[69] Others have transformed visual field sensitivities in decibels to a linear scale.[1,78] It is possible that transforming structural or functional measurements to a common domain might be useful for subsequent Bayesian analyses, however, the purpose of these studies has been primarily to examine the relationship between structural and functional tests and not to combine the results in a single model. The use of these methods to explore the relationship between structure and function is discussed elsewhere in this consensus statement.

3.6.3.3. Method #3: Combined structure-function index

The combined structure-function index (CSFI) has been proposed by Medeiros and colleagues as a method of combining results from structural and functional tests.[22] The CSFI is an estimate of the percentage of retinal ganglion cells lost compared to that expected for an age-matched healthy eye, *i.e.*, an eye with a CSFI of 25% would have an estimated retinal ganglion cell count 25% less than that expected for age.

The estimate of retinal ganglion cells is derived from structural and functional tests using a series of formulas originally derived from studies of experimental glaucoma in monkeys but subsequently validated in human clinical cohorts.[22,1] The models relate SAP sensitivity measurements to histological numbers of retinal ganglion cells as a function of retinal eccentricity with the experimental results then translated to human clinical perimetry.[1] The formulas allow retinal ganglion cell numbers to be estimated from perimetric threshold sensitivity values. The relationship between OCT RNFL thickness and histological retinal ganglion cell counts was also examined, and taking into account the effect of disease severity on neuronal and non-neuronal constituents of the RNFL, formulas were developed for estimating numbers of retinal ganglion cell axons from OCT.

The ability to estimate retinal ganglion cell numbers from OCT and SAP provides a common unit for combining structural and functional information.

The CSFI combines estimates using a weighting to account for the differences in performance of OCT and SAP at different stages of disease, assigning greater importance to OCT in early disease and SAP in moderate to advanced disease, where there is a floor in structural measurements.[15,19]

The CSFI has shown good ability to differentiate glaucomatous and healthy eyes, performing better than isolated measures of structure and function.[22] In a study of 333 glaucomatous and 165 healthy eyes, the CSFI achieved an area under the receiver operating curve (AROC) of 0.94, which was significantly better than OCT RNFL thickness (AROC = 0.92, $P = 0.008$), SAP MD (AROC = 0.88, $P < 0.001$) and SAP VFI (AUC = 0.89, $P < 0.001$).[22] A subgroup analysis of 38 eyes with pre-perimetric glaucoma, defined by progressive optic disc changes on stereo-photographs, showed the CSFI to maintain good ability to differentiate health and disease with an AROC of 0.85. The CSFI also performed well and better than OCT to stage disease severity. It was also shown to be useful for predicting glaucoma (repeatable abnormal visual fields or progressive optic disc changes) in glaucoma suspects, performing better than isolated structural or functional measurements.[79]

Advantages

A potential advantage of the CSFI is that by incorporating a weighting for disease severity it can draw on the differing strengths of structural and functional tests at different stages of the disease process. Estimation of retinal ganglion cell numbers is also an intuitive unit for expressing severity of glaucomatous damage.

Limitations

The CSFI has potential limitations, such as the fact that the combined estimates of retinal ganglion cell count have not been validated using human clinical data. However, it should be noted that this might be irrelevant in the context of applying the index for diagnosis and assessment of disease progression. In fact, there is considerable disagreement between RNFL thickness measurements given by different OCT devices and histological RNFL thickness measurements and this does not preclude the use of OCT in clinical practice.

References

1. Harwerth RS, Wheat JL, Fredette MJ, Anderson DR. Linking structure and function in glaucoma. Prog Retin Eye Res 2010;29(4):249-271.
2. Hood DC, Kardon RH. A framework for comparing structural and functional measures of glaucomatous damage. Prog Retin Eye Res 2007;26(6):688-7
3. Drasdo N, Millican CL, Katholi CR, Curcio CA. The length of Henle fibers in the human retina and a model of ganglion receptive field density in the visual field. Vision Res 2007;47:2901-2911.
4. Malik R, Swanson WH, Garway-Heath DF. 'Structure-function relationship' in glaucoma: past thinking and current concepts. Clin Experiment Ophthalmol 2012;40:369-380.
5. Quigley HA, Dunkelberger GR, Green WR. Retinal ganglion cell atrophy correlated with automated perimetry in human eyes with glaucoma. Am J Ophthalmol 1989;107:453-464.
6. Medeiros FA, Alencar LM, Zangwill LM, Bowd C, Sample PA, Weinreb RN. Prediction of functional loss in glaucoma from progressive optic disc damage. Arch Ophthalmol 2009;127(10):1250-12doi: 10.1001/archophthalmol.2009.276.
7. Gordon MO, Beiser JA, Brandt JD, et al. The Ocular Hypertension Treatment Study: baseline factors that predict the onset of primary open-angle glaucoma. 2002;120 (6):714-720.
8. Miglior S, Zeyen T, Pfeiffer N, et al. Results of the European Glaucoma Prevention Study. Ophthalmology 2005;112:366-375.
9. Garway-Heath DF, Poinoosawmy D, Fitzke FW, Hitchings RA. Mapping the visual field to the optic disc in normal tension glaucoma eyes. Ophthalmology 2000;107(10):1809-1815.
10. Harwerth RS, Carter-Dawson L, Shen F, et al. Ganglion cell losses underlying visual field defects from experimental glaucoma. Invest Ophthalmol Vis Sci 1999;40:2242-2250.
11. Swanson WH, Felius J, Pan F. Perimetric defects and ganglion cell damage: interpreting linear relations using a two-stage neural model. Invest Ophthalmol Vis Sci 2004;45(2):466-472.
12. Drasdo N, Mortlock KE, North RV. Ganglion cell loss and dysfunction: relationship to perimetric sensitivity. Optom Vis Sci 2008;85(11):1036-10doi: 10.1097/OPX.0b013e31818b94af. Erratum in: Optom Vis Sci. 2008Dec;85(12):1205.
13. Pan F, Swanson WH. A cortical pooling model of spatial summation for perimetric stimuli. J Vis 2006;6(11):1159-1171.
14. Medeiros FA, Zangwill LM, Bowd C, Mansouri K, Weinreb RN. The structure and function relationship in glaucoma: implications for detection of progression and measurement of rates of change. Invest Ophthalmol Vis Sci 2012;53(11):6939-69doi: 10.1167/iovs.12-10345.
15. Medeiros FA, Zangwill LM, Anderson DR, et al. Estimating the rate of retinal ganglion cell loss in glaucoma. Am J Ophthalmol 2012;154(5):814-824.
16. Ventura LM, Porciatti V. Restoration of Retinal Ganglion Cell Function in Early Glaucoma after Intraocular Pressure Reduction. Ophthalmology 2005;112(1):20-27.
17. Sun H, Swanson WH, Arvidson B, Dul MW. Assessment of contrast gain signature in inferred magnocellular and parvocellular pathways in patients with glaucoma. Vision Res 2008; 48(26):2633-26
18. Sihota R, Sony P, Gupta V, Dada T, Singh R. Diagnostic capability of optical coherence tomography in evaluating the degree of glaucomatous retinal nerve fiber damage. Invest Ophthalmol Vis Sci 2006;47(5):2006-2010.
19. Mwanza JC, Budenz DL, Warren JL, et al. Retinal nerve fibre layer thickness floor and corresponding functional loss in glaucoma. Br J Ophthalmol 2015;99(6):732-7doi: 10.1136/bjophthalmol-2014-3057Epub 2014 Dec 9.

20. Lamparter J, Russell RA, Zhu H, et al. The influence of intersubject variability in ocular anatomical variables on the mapping of retinal locations to the retinal nerve fiber layer and optic nerve head. Invest Ophthalmol Vis Sci 2013;54(9):6074-60doi: 10.1167/iovs.13-11902.
21. Jansonius NM, Nevalainen J, Selig B, et al. A mathematical description of nerve fiber bundle trajectories and their variability in the human retina. Vision Res 2009;49(17):2157-2163.
22. Medeiros FA, Lisboa R, Weinreb RN, et al. A combined index of structure and function for staging glaucomatous damage. Arch Ophthalmol 2012;130:1107-1116.
23. Jansonius NM, Schiefer J, Nevalainen J, Paetzold J, Schiefer U. A mathematical model for describing the retinal nerve fiber bundle trajectories in the human eye: average course, variability, and influence of refraction, optic disc size and optic disc position. Exp Eye Res 2012;105:70-78.
24. Denniss J, McKendrick AM, Turpin A. An anatomically-customisable computational model relating the visual field to the optic nerve head in individual eyes. Invest Ophthalmol Vis Sci. 2012;53(11):6981-6990.
25. Ferreras A, Pablo LE, Garway-Heath DF, Fogagnolo P, García-Feijoo J. Mapping standard automated perimetry to the peripapillary retinal nerve fiber layer in glaucoma. Invest Ophthalmol Vis Sci 2008;49:3018-3025.
26. Gardiner SK, Johnson CA, Cioffi GA. Evaluation of the structure-function relationship in glaucoma. Invest Ophthalmol Vis Sci 2005;46(10)3712-37
27. Turpin A, Sampson GP, McKendrick AM. Combining ganglion cell topology and data of patients with glaucoma to determine a structure-function map. Invest Ophthalmol Vis Sci 2009;50(7):3249-3256.
28. Erler NS, Bryan SR, Eilers PHC, Lesaffre EM, Lemij HG, Vermeer KA. Optimizing Structure–Function Relationship by Maximizing Correspondence Between Glaucomatous Visual Fields and Mathematical Retinal Nerve Fiber Models, Invest Ophthalmol Vis Sci 2014;55: 2350-2357.
29. Denniss J, Turpin A, Tanabe F, Matsumoto C, McKendrick AM. Structure-Function Mapping: Variability and Conviction in Tracing Retinal Nerve Fibre Bundles and Comparison to a Computational Model. Invest Ophthalmol Vis Sci 2014a;55(2):728-736.
30. Chauhan BC, Burgoyne CF. From Clinical Examination of the Optic Disc to Clinical Assessment of the Optic Nerve Head: A Paradigm Change. Am J Ophthalmol 2013;156:218-227.
31. Amini N, Nowroozizadeh S, Cirineo N, et al. Influence of the disc-fovea angle on limits of RNFL variability and glaucoma discrimination. Invest Ophthalmol Vis Sci 2014;55:7332-7342.
32. Chauhan BC, Sharpe GA, Hutchinson DM. Imaging of the temporal raphe with optical coherence tomography. Ophthalmology 2014;121(11):2287-2288.
33. Tanabe F, Matsumoto C, Okuyama S, et al. Imaging of temporal retinal nerve fiber layer with transverse section analysis. Invest Ophthalmol Vis Sci 2014;55:901.
34. Huang G, Luo T, Gast TJ, et al. Imaging glaucomatous damage across the temporal raphe. Invest Ophthalmol Vis Sci 2015;56(6):3496-3504.
35. Denniss J, Turpin A, McKendrick AM. Individualised structure-function mapping for glaucoma: practical constraints on map resolution of clinical and research applications. Invest Ophthalmol Vis Sci 2014b;55(3):1985-1993.
36. Ganeshrao SB, Turpin A, Denniss J, McKendrick AM. Enhancing structure-function correlations in glaucoma with customised spatial mapping. Ophthalmology 2015;122(8):1695-1705.
37. Sjöstrand J, Popovic Z, Conradi N, Marshall J. Morphometric study of the displacement of retinal ganglion cells subserving cones within the human fovea. Graefes Arch Clin Exp Ophthalmol 1999;237:1014-1023.

38. Watson AB. A formula for human retinal ganglion cell receptive field density as a function of visual field location. J Vis 2014;14:1-17.
39. Hood DC, Raza AS, de Moraes CGV, Liebmann JM, Ritch R. Glaucomatous damage of the macula. Prog Retin Eye Res 2013;32:1-21.
40. Hood DC, Raza AS. On improving the use of OCT imaging for detecting glaucomatous damage. Br J Ophthalmol 2014;98:ii1-ii9.
41. Tick S, Rossant F, Ghorbel I, et al. Foveal Shape and Structure in a Normal Population. Invest Ophthalmol Vis Sci 2011;52(8):5105-5110.
42. Turpin A, Chen S, Sepulveda JA, McKendrick AM. Customising structure-function displacements in the macula for individual differences. Invest Ophthalmol Vis Sci 2015;56(10):5984-5989.
43. Garway-Heath DF, Hitchings RA. Sources of bias in studies of optic disc and retinal nerve fibre layer morphology. Br J Ophthalmol 1998;82:986.
44. Rao HL, Yadav RK, Addepalli UK, et al. Reference Standard Test and the Diagnostic Ability of Spectral Domain Optical Coherence Tomography in Glaucoma. J Glaucoma 2015;24:e151-156.
45. Sample PA, Medeiros FA, Racette L, et al. Identifying glaucomatous vision loss with visual-function-specific perimetry in the diagnostic innovations in glaucoma study. Invest Ophthalmol Vis Sci 2006;47:3381-3389.
46. Leung CK, Cheung CY, Weinreb RN, et al. Retinal nerve fiber layer imaging with spectral-domain optical coherence tomography: a variability and diagnostic performance study. Ophthalmology 2009;116:1257-1263, 63 e1-2.
47. Moreno-Montanes J, Olmo N, Alvarez A, et al. Cirrus high-definition optical coherence tomography compared with Stratus optical coherence tomography in glaucoma diagnosis. Invest Ophthalmol Vis Sci 2010;51:335-343.
48. Rao HL, Zangwill LM, Weinreb RN, et al. Comparison of different spectral domain optical coherence tomography scanning areas for glaucoma diagnosis. Ophthalmology 2010;117:1692-1699, 9 e1.
49. Kerrigan-Baumrind LA, Quigley HA, Pease ME, et al. Number of ganglion cells in glaucoma eyes compared with threshold visual field tests in the same persons. Invest Ophthalmol Vis Sci 2000;41:741-748.
50. Sommer A, Katz J, Quigley HA, et al. Clinically detectable nerve fiber atrophy precedes the onset of glaucomatous field loss. Arch Ophthalmol 1991;109:77-83.
51. Kuang TM, Zhang C, Zangwill LM, et al. Estimating Lead Time Gained by Optical Coherence Tomography in Detecting Glaucoma before Development of Visual Field Defects. Ophthalmology 2015;122:2002-2009.
52. Keltner JL, Johnson CA, Anderson DR, et al. The association between glaucomatous visual fields and optic nerve head features in the Ocular Hypertension Treatment Study. Ophthalmology 2006;113:1603-1612.
53. Heijl A, Leske MC, Bengtsson B, et al. Reduction of intraocular pressure and glaucoma progression: results from the Early Manifest Glaucoma Trial. Arch Ophthalmol 2002;120:1268-1279.
54. Tatham AJ, Medeiros FA, Zangwill LM, Weinreb RN. Strategies to improve early diagnosis in glaucoma. Prog Brain Res 2015;221:103-133.
55. Harwerth RS, Quigley HA. Visual field defects and retinal ganglion cell losses in patients with glaucoma. Arch Ophthalmol 2006;124:853-859.

56. Chauhan BC, Garway-Heath DF, Goñi FJ, et al. Practical recommendations for measuring rates of visual field change in glaucoma. Br J Ophthalmol 2008;92(4):569-5doi: 10.1136/bjo.2007.1350Epub 2008 Jan Review.
57. Hood DC, Raza AS, De Moraes CG, et al. Evaluation of a One-Page Report to Aid in Detecting Glaucomatous Damage. Transl Vis Sci Technol 2014;3(6):8.
58. Wong EN, Mackey DA, Morgan WH, Chen FK. Intersession test-retest variability of conventional and novel parameters using the MP-1 microperimeter. Clin Ophthalmol 2016;10:29-42.
59. Sato S, Hirooka K, Baba T, et al. Correlation between the ganglion cell-inner plexiform layer thickness measured with cirrus HD-OCT and macular visual field sensitivity measured with microperimetry. Invest Ophthalmol Vis Sci 2013;54(4):3046-3051.
60. Rossetti L, Digiuni M, Rosso A, et al. Compass: clinical evaluation of a new instrument for the diagnosis of glaucoma. PloS one 2015;10(3):e0122157.
61. Hood DC, Raza AS, de Moraes CG, et al. Initial arcuate defects within the central 10 degrees in glaucoma. Invest Ophthalmol Vis Sci 2011;52(2):940-946.
62. Ehrlich AC, Raza AS, Ritch R, Hood DC. Modifying the Conventional Visual Field Test Pattern to Improve the Detection of Early Glaucomatous Defects in the Central 10 degrees. Transl Vis Sci Technol 2014;3(6):6.
63. Chen S, McKendrick AM, Turpin A. Choosing two points to add to the 24-2 pattern to better describe macular visual field damage due to glaucoma. Brit J Ophthalmol 2015;99(9):1236-1239.
64. Kass MA, Heuer DK, Higginbotham EJ, et al. The Ocular Hypertension Treatment Study: a randomized trial determines that topical ocular hypotensive medication delays or prevents the onset of primary open-angle glaucoma. Arch Ophthalmol 2002;120(6):701-713; discussion 829-830.
65. Schiefer U, Papageorgiou E, Sample PA, et al. Spatial pattern of glaucomatous visual field loss obtained with regionally condensed stimulus arrangements. Invest Ophthalmol Vis Sci 2010;51(11):5685-5689.
66. Chong LX, McKendrick AM, Ganeshrao SB, Turpin A. Customized, automated stimulus location choice for assessment of visual field defects. Invest Ophthalmol Vis Sci 2014;55(5):3265-3274.
67. Denniss J, McKendrick AM, Turpin A. Towards Patient-Tailored Perimetry: Automated Perimetry Can Be Improved by Seeding Procedures With Patient-Specific Structural Information. Transl Vis Sci Technol 2013;2(4):3.
68. Ganeshrao SB, McKendrick AM, Denniss J, Turpin A. A perimetric test procedure that uses structural information. Optometry and vision science: official publication of the Amer Acad Optom 2015;92(1):70-82.
69. Zhu H, Crabb DP, Schlottmann PG, et al. Predicting visual function from the measurements of retinal nerve fiber layer structure. Invest Ophthalmol Vis Sci 2010;51(11):5657-5666.
70. Sugimoto K, Murata H, Hirasawa H, et al. Cross-sectional study: Does combining optical coherence tomography measurements using the 'Random Forest' decision tree classifier improve the prediction of the presence of perimetric deterioration in glaucoma suspects? BMJ Open 2013;3(10):e0031doi: 10.1136/bmjopen-2013-003114.
71. Deng L, Demirel S, Gardiner SK. Reducing variability in visual field assessment for glaucoma through filtering that combines structural and functional information. Invest Ophthalmol Vis Sci 2014;55(7):4593-4602.
72. Asaoka R, Russell RA, Malik R, Crabb DP, Garway-Heath DF. A novel distribution of visual field test points to improve the correlation between structure-function measurements. Invest Ophthalmol Vis Sci 2012;53(13):8396-8404.

73. Artes PH, Chauhan BC. Longitudinal changes in the visual field and optic disc in glaucoma. Prog Retin Eye Res 2005;24:333-354.
74. Russell RA, Malik R, Chauhan BC, et al. Improved estimates of visual field progression using Bayesian linear regression to integrate structural information in patients with ocular hypertension. Invest Ophthalmol Vis Sci 2012;53:2760-2769.
75. Thomas R, Mengersen K, Parikh RS, et al. Enter the reverend: introduction to and application of Bayes' theorem in clinical ophthalmology. Clin Experiment Ophthalmol 2011;39:865-870.
76. Medeiros FA, Zangwill LM, Girkin CA, et al. Combining structural and functional measurements to improve estimates of rates of glaucomatous progression. Am J Ophthalmol 2012;153:1197-1205.e1.
77. Medeiros FA, Leite MT, Zangwill LM, et al. Combining structural and functional measurements to improve detection of glaucoma progression using Bayesian hierarchical models. Invest Ophthalmol Vis Sci 2011;52:5794-5803.
78. Garway-Heath DF, Caprioli J, Fitzke FW, et al. Scaling the hill of vision: the physiological relationship between light sensitivity and ganglion cell numbers. Invest Ophthalmol Vis Sci 2000;41:1774-1782.
79. Meira-Freitas D, Lisboa R, Tatham A, et al. Predicting progression in glaucoma suspects with longitudinal estimates of retinal ganglion cell counts. Invest Ophthalmol Vis Sci 2013;54:4174-4183.

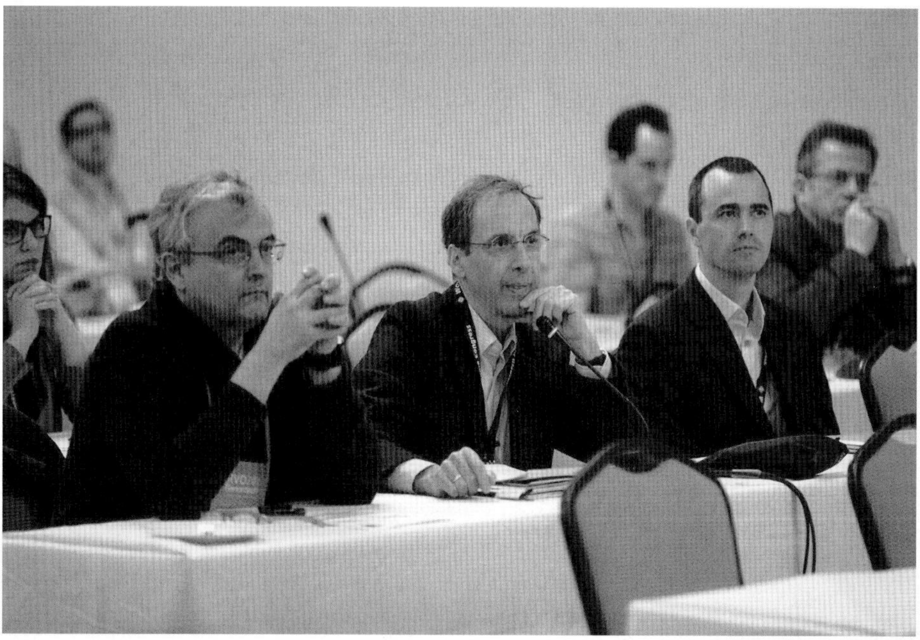

Stefano Gandolfi, Norbert Pfeiffer and Andrew Tatham

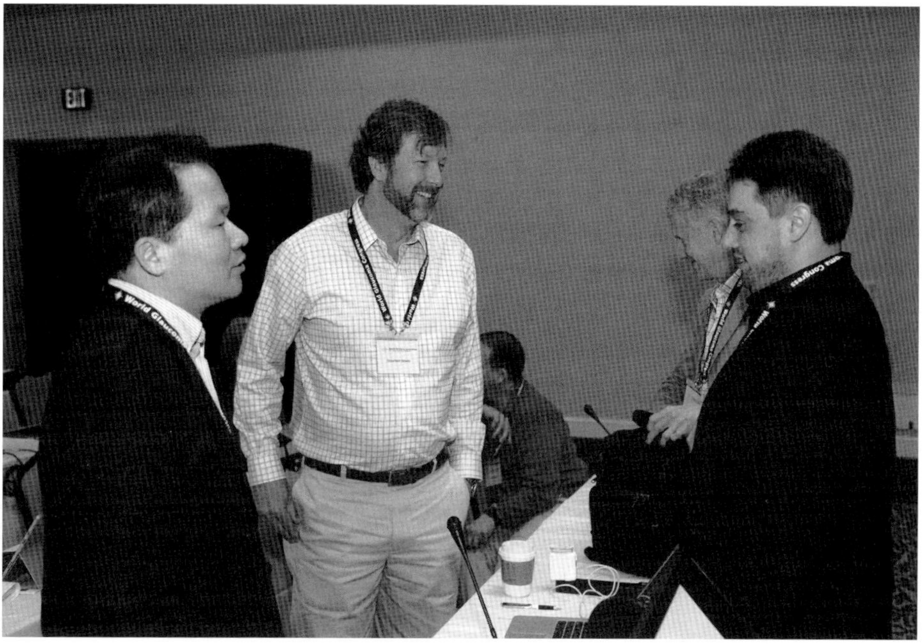

Tae Woo Kim and Crawford Downs

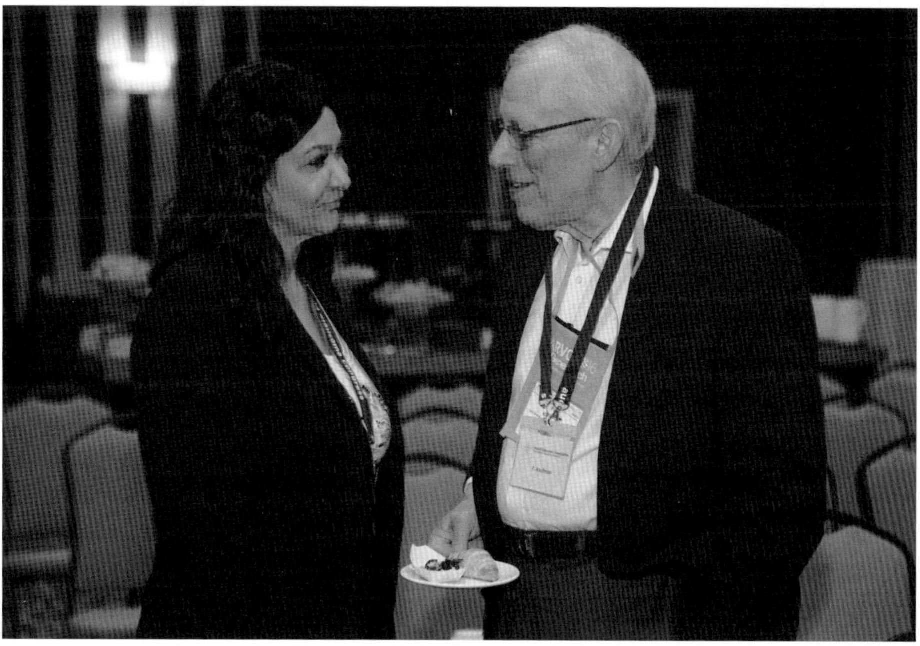

Neeru Gupta and Paul Kaufman

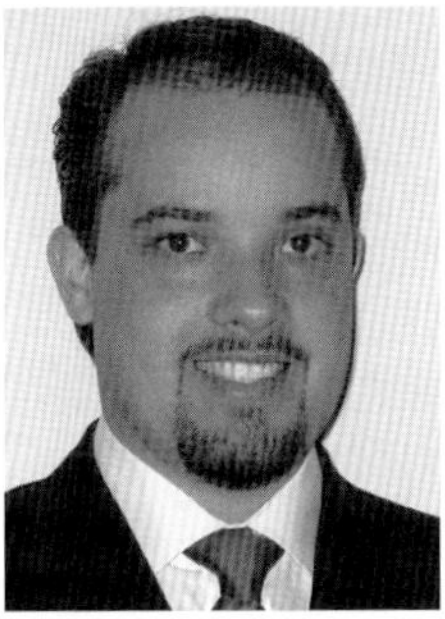

Felipe A. Medeiros

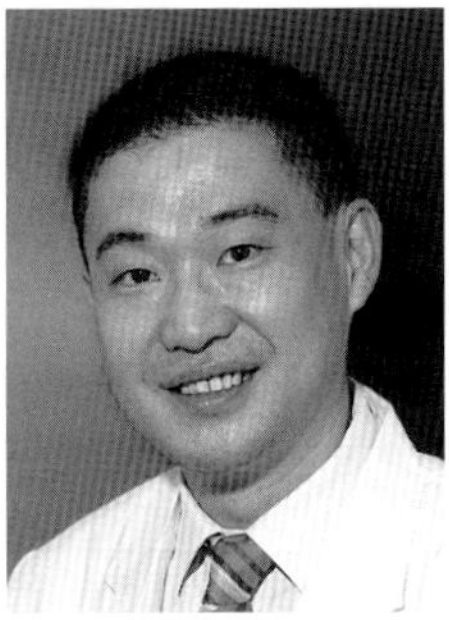

Mingguang He

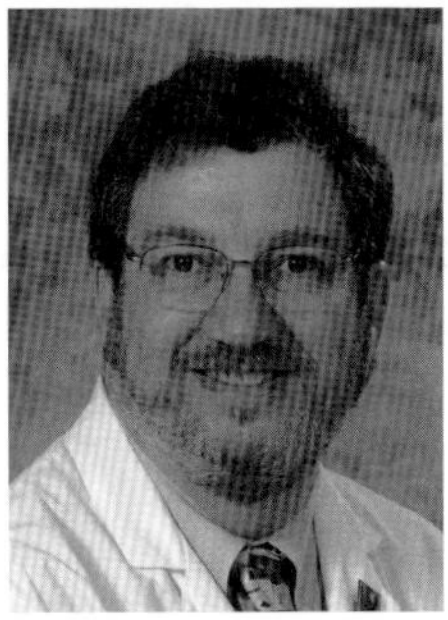

James Brandt

4. RISK FACTORS (OCULAR)

Section leader: Felipe A. Medeiros
Section co-leaders: Mingguang He, James Brandt
Contributors: Tin Aung, Eytan Blumenthal, Anne Louise Coleman, Jonathan Crowston, Gustavo de Moraes, Crawford Downs, Robert Fechtner, Panayiota Founti, Christopher Girkin, Neeru Gupta, Alon Harris, Henry D. Jampel, Vijaya Lingam, Christopher Leung, Steve Mansberger, Stefano Miglior, Augusto Paranhos, Louis R. Pasquale, Remo Susanna Jr., Ningli Wang

Consensus statements

1. Although POAG may develop at any IOP, there is strong evidence supporting higher mean intraocular pressure during follow-up as a risk factor for development and progression of glaucomatous damage.
   Comments: There is insufficient evidence and further studies are needed to elucidate which IOP parameter(s) (mean, peak and/or fluctuation, area under IOP curve, etc.) is most important in determining risk of glaucoma development or progression.
   There is insufficient evidence implicating IOP fluctuations as an independent risk factor for glaucoma development or progression.
2. Low ocular perfusion pressure (OPP) (the difference between systemic blood pressure and intraocular pressure) is associated with increased prevalence of open-angle glaucoma in cross-sectional studies.
   Comments: The value of OPP monitoring in daily clinical practice is not established.
   Due to the intrinsic relationship between OPP and IOP, it is difficult to establish an independent contribution of OPP as a risk factor for the development of glaucoma.
3. There is insufficient evidence supporting the role of provocative tests, such as the water-drinking test, as providing independent contribution to assess risk of glaucoma development and progression.
   Comment: Prospective longitudinal studies are necessary to clarify whether

Diagnosis of Primary Open Angle Glaucoma, pp 127-158
Edited by Robert N. Weinreb, David Garway-Heath, Christopher Leung, Felipe Medeiros, Jeffrey Liebmann

the water-drinking provocative test can provide additional information over office-based IOP measurements in establishing risk of glaucoma development or progression.

4. There is strong evidence supporting the role of central corneal thickness (CCT) as an important predictive factor for glaucoma development in ocular hypertensives and glaucoma suspects. Baseline CCT measurements should be obtained in patients suspected of having glaucoma.

   Comments: Algorithms to correct IOP based on CCT measurements are not recommended for routine use in clinical practice.

   There is insufficient evidence to conclude whether or not CCT is a true independent risk factor for glaucoma development or progression, or whether its effect is related to a tonometric artifact.

   There is no evidence that serial CCT measurements have value in clinical evaluation glaucoma.

5. There is strong evidence implicating lower corneal hysteresis as a risk factor for glaucoma development and progression.

   Comments: There is insufficient evidence about the mechanisms by which corneal hysteresis is associated with risk of glaucoma progression.

6. Existing evidence suggests that individuals with myopia have an increased risk of developing open angle glaucoma, with the risk being greater for people with high myopia.

   Comments: Diagnosis of glaucoma among myopic eyes can be challenging. Confirmed evidence of glaucomatous progression from a well-defined baseline is important for a correct diagnosis in many myopic individuals.

7. Disc hemorrhage is associated with increased risk of developing glaucoma and it is a marker for glaucomatous progression.

   Comment: Consideration of treatment escalation or closer follow-up should be given for patients presenting with optic disc hemorrhages.

8. Predictive models (risk calculators) may provide objective assessment of individual risk and their use should be considered in patients suspected of having glaucoma.

   Comment: Current validated risk calculators apply only to OHT patients. Moreover, they do not include all known risk factors.

4.1. Intraocular Pressure (IOP)

Intraocular pressure (IOP) has been consistently demonstrated to be associated with development and progression of glaucoma. Below we summarize some of the evidence currently available with regard to IOP parameters and risk of glaucoma development and progression.

4.1.1. Mean IOP as a risk factor for glaucoma development

There is strong evidence from several clinical trials to support higher mean IOP as a risk factor for development of glaucoma, as well as for progression of disease in individuals with manifest glaucoma. In the OHTS, EGPS, EMGT, AGIS, the Canadian Glaucoma Study, DIGS and UKGTS each mmHg of increased mean IOP was associated with an increased risk for progression of 10-25%.

The **Ocular Hypertension Treatment Study (OHTS)** has provided strong evidence with regard to the role of IOP as a risk factor for development of glaucoma. In the OHTS, 1636 ocular hypertensive patients were randomized to either observation or treatment and followed for a median time of 72 months. Ocular hypertension was defined based on the presence of qualifying IOP between 24 mmHg and 32 mmHg in one eye and between 21 mmHg and 32 mmHg in the other eye, gonioscopically open angles, normal visual fields and normal optic discs.[1] Participants randomized to medication began treatment to achieve a target IOP of 24 mmHg or less and a minimum of 20% reduction in IOP from the average of the qualifying IOP and IOP at the baseline randomization visit. At baseline, mean IOP was 24.9 ± 2.6 mmHg and 24.9 ± 2.7 mmHg in the treated and observation groups, respectively. The average IOP reduction in the treated group was 22.5% ± 9.9% compared to 4.0% ± 11.6% in the observation group. At 60 months, the cumulative probability of developing POAG was 4.4% in the medication group compared to 9.5% in the observation group, which translates into a 54% relative reduction in the risk of developing POAG with treatment. In the analysis of baseline predictive factors for development of POAG, 1 mmHg higher baseline IOP was associated with a 10% higher risk of developing POAG during follow-up, after adjustment for other predictive factors in a multivariate model.[2] For this calculation, baseline IOP was calculated from four to six baseline IOP measurements per eye.

The **European Glaucoma Prevention Study (EGPS)**[3] was also designed to investigate whether the onset of POAG can be prevented or delayed in ocular

however, the untreated baseline median intraocular pressure was not significantly related to the rate of progression. According to the CNTGS authors,[13] this discrepancy could be potentially explained by the fact that the rate of progression could be related not to the absolute level of IOP, but to the amount by which the IOP exceeds the damage threshold of a particular individual. The amount of excess could be unrelated to the presenting baseline IOP in NTG patients. Therapeutic lowering of the pressure would reduce the IOP relative to the damage threshold and slow the rate of progression.

Other prospective clinical trials have also provided evidence that IOP is a risk factor for glaucoma progression. However, it is important to note that these trials were not originally designed to specifically address the relationship between IOP reduction and glaucoma progression. The **Advanced Glaucoma Intervention Study (AGIS)**[14] was a long-term study designed to evaluate the clinical course of medically uncontrolled OAG by two surgical treatment sequences. Of 591 patients, 789 eyes were randomized to a treatment sequence of (1) argon laser trabeculoplasty, trabeculectomy and trabeculectomy (ATT); or (2) trabeculectomy, argon laser trabeculoplasty and trabeculectomy (TAA). To be eligible for the AGIS, eyes had to meet specific criteria consisting of combinations of uncontrolled IOP with medications, glaucomatous visual field defect and/or optic disc damage. During follow-up, surgical interventions were supplemented by medical therapy with the goal of reducing IOP to less than 18 mmHg. One of the AGIS reports[14] examined the relationship between control of IOP and visual field deterioration. In the so-called Associative Analysis, eyes were divided according to the percent of visits for which the eye presented IOP less than 18 mmHg. Eyes were assigned to one of four categories: 100% (group A), 75% to less than 100% (group B), 50% to less than 75% (group C) and 0 to less than 50% (group D). The mean IOP over the six years of follow-up was 12.3 mmHg in group A, 14.7 mmHg in group B, 16.9 mmHg in group C and 20.2 mmHg in group D. Eyes in group A had mean changes from baseline in visual field defect score close to zero. Patients in groups B, C and D had progressively more changes in visual field compared to group A. At 7 years of follow-up, eyes in group D had an estimated worsening of 1.93 (95% CI: 0.82-3.05) units of visual field defect score compared to eyes in group A, after adjustment for potentially confounding covariates.

In the analysis of predictive factors for progression of visual field loss in the AGIS, each 1 mmHg higher mean IOP level at the first 18 months of follow-up was associated with a 0.10 increase in visual field defect score during the rest of follow-up ($P = 0.002$), after adjusting for race, assigned intervention sequence, age, diabetes, gender, reference IOP and reference visual field defect score.[14]

It is important to note that although AGIS results support a relationship between IOP and rate of glaucoma progression, the secondary analyses described above involved non-randomized groups that had potentially imbalanced covariate values. However, results were consistent even after adjustment for potentially confounding covariates using statistical methods.

The **Collaborative Initial Glaucoma Treatment Study (CIGTS)**[15] randomized 607 patients with newly diagnosed OAG to medical versus surgical treatment. Each patient was assigned a target IOP that was a function of baseline IOP and a reference visual field, so that patients with more severe disease were required to have more IOP lowering. Average MD of baseline visual fields was -5 dB. Patients assigned to the medical arm were treated with IOP-lowering treatments at the discretion of the treating physician, whereas patients assigned to the surgical arm underwent trabeculectomy (with 5-FU at the discretion of the surgeon). Average baseline IOPs were 27 mmHg and 28 mmHg in the surgical and medical group, respectively. IOP was reduced, on average, by approximately 48% and 35% in the surgical and medical group, respectively. Visual fields were graded using a defined protocol (increasing scores reflecting increasing VF loss and ranging from 0 to 20). Both groups had, on average, minimal changes in visual field scores over time. Repeated measures analysis of variance modeling adjusting for visual field score at baseline, age, race, gender and diagnosis showed that initial surgery resulted in 0.36 unit worse visual field score than initial medical treatment ($P = 0.003$); however, when the influence of cataract was included in the model, the difference decrease to 0.28 units ($P = 0.07$). The greater lowering of mean IOP in the surgically treated group apparently was of no further benefit in CIGTS patients. However, a subsequent analysis of longer-term results did reveal a better outcome for the surgical group in a subset of subjects with a greater degree of initial visual field loss.[16]

When contrasted to the EMGT, however, results from the CIGTS seem to indicate that a substantial reduction of IOP decreases the rate of glaucoma progression. Both studies included patients with relatively early glaucoma at baseline (average MD was -4dB in EMGT and -5dB in CIGTS), although different methods were used to assess visual field progression. In the medically treated patients in the CIGTS an IOP reduction of approximately 35% resulted in no net visual field loss, whereas in the EMGT, an average IOP reduction of 25% resulted in 45% of the patients developing visual field loss over time. Whereas in the CIGTS, medical treatment was aggressive to reduce the IOP to the target level, a fixed treatment protocol was used in the EMGT. The mean ± SD IOP reduction from baseline IOP in the EMGT was -4.5 ± 3.4 mmHg, that is, assuming a normal distribution, approximately 25% of the patients had IOP reduction less than 2 mmHg with treatment and approximately 35% had IOP reduction less than 3 mmHg. The suboptimal IOP reduction in many patients is likely to be related to the high rate of visual field progression in the EMGT.

The **United Kingdom Glaucoma Treatment Study** was the first prospective randomized placebo-controlled clinical trial to evaluate the efficacy of intraocular pressure reduction in preventing glaucoma progression. In the UKGTS, 516 individuals were enrolled between Dec 1, 2006, and March 16, 2010. Baseline mean intraocular pressure was 19.6 mmHg (SD 4.6) in patients randomized to the latanoprost group and 20.1 mmHg (4.8) in the control group. At 24 months of follow-up, mean reduction in intraocular pressure was 3.8 mmHg (4.0) in the latanoprost group compared to 0.9 mmHg (3.8) in the placebo group. Visual field preservation was significantly longer in the latanoprost group compared to the placebo group, with an adjusted hazard ratio (HR) 0.44 (95% CI 0.28–0.69; p = 0.0003). When risk per 1 mmHg IOP reduction is calculated, each 1 mmHg higher mean IOP translated into approximately 24% greater risk.

4.1.2. IOP fluctuations as a risk factor for glaucoma

IOP is a dynamic parameter with a circadian rhythm and spontaneous changes. Although variations in IOP are commonly noticed, they are not well characterized and are often underappreciated in the management of glaucoma patients. These variations are the result of complex interactions between external stimuli and intrinsic biological IOP rhythm. IOP fluctuations of as much as 4-5 mmHg in healthy individuals and, substantially higher, in some glaucoma patients have been reported.

Despite several reports regarding the clinical relevance of IOP fluctuation in POAG, as of today there are limited and generally inconsistent results concerning the actual risk for the onset or progression of POAG associated with either 24 hour fluctuation or long-term variability.[17] This is in part related to difficulties in continuously assessing IOP over time.

4.1.2.1. Long-term IOP variation as a risk factor for glaucoma

The EGPS did not find long-term IOP variation to be significantly associated with the risk of conversion from ocular hypertension to glaucoma. Long-term IOP variation was also calculated as the standard deviation of mean IOP over time. In the univariate analysis long-term IOP fluctuation had a HR = 0.87 per 1 mmHg higher; 95% CI: 0.70-1.09; p = 0.23). In the multivariate model, adjusting by inter-current factors such as disc hemorrhage, diabetes, systemic hypertension, systemic diuretics, systemic ACE inhibitors, treatment arm and all the baseline predictive factors (age, CCT, PSD, vertical c/d ratio, vertical c/d ratio asymmetry), mean IOP was significantly associated with glaucoma conversion (adjusted HR = 1.12 per 1 mmHg higher; 95% CI: 1.03 to 1.22; p = 0.007).[18]

A report from the DIGS by Medeiros *et al.*[19] involved 126 ocular hypertensive patients followed for an average time of seven years. They did not find long-term IOP variation to be significantly associated with the risk of conversion from ocular hypertension to glaucoma. All patients in the study had high intraocular pressure (> 22 mmHg), normal optic discs and normal visual fields at baseline. Conversion to glaucoma was defined based on the development of repeatable visual field loss or progressive change to the optic disc as evaluated by stereophotographs. Forty eyes of 31 subjects developed POAG during follow-up. Long-term IOP variation was calculated as the standard deviation of IOP measurements over time. In a multivariate model adjusting for age, CCT, PSD, vertical cup/disc ratio and mean IOP, long-term IOP variation was not significantly associated with glaucoma conversion (adjusted HR = 1.08 per 1 mmHg higher; 95% CI: 0.79 to 1.48; P = 0.620). Mean IOP was significantly associated with glaucoma conversion (adjusted HR = 1.20 per 1 mmHg higher; 95% CI: 1.06 to 1.36; P = 0.005).

In the **Malmö Ocular Hypertension Study**, Bengtsson and Heijl[20] followed high-risk ocular hypertensive patients for ten years as part of a prospective investigation in order to compare the rates of development of glaucomatous visual field loss in patients treated with timolol compared to placebo. Patients were followed every three months with Goldmann tonometry measurements obtained at 8:00 am, 11:30 am and 3:30 pm. No association was found between parameters measuring long-term IOP variation and the risk of glaucoma development.

As part of the EMGT, Bengtsson *et al.*[21] did not find long-term IOP variation to be associated with visual field progression. The definition of long-term IOP variation was also based on the standard deviation of IOP measurements over time. However, IOP measurements were only included up to the date of progression (for progressors) or last follow-up visit (for non-progressors). The analysis involved 255 patients with a median follow-up time of eight years. Mean long-term IOP fluctuations were 2.02 mmHg and 1.78 mmHg in patients who progressed and in patients who did not progressed, respectively. In a multivariate Cox regression model, IOP variation was not a significant risk factor for progression (adjusted HR = 1.0; 95% CI: 0.81-1.24; P = 0.999). The model adjusted for mean IOP, age, baseline IOP, presence of exfoliation, severity of visual field loss at baseline and whether one or both eyes were eligible for the study. Mean IOP was significantly associated with risk of progressive visual field loss. Each 1 mmHg higher mean IOP was associated with 11% increase in risk. Similar results were identified when treated and control patients were analyzed separately.

In a post-hoc analysis of AGIS data, Nouri-Mahdavi *et al.*[22] found that long-term IOP fluctuations were a statistically significant risk factor associated with visual field progression. Long-term IOP variation was calculated as the standard deviation of all available IOP measurements during follow-up, after the initial surgical procedure. In a multivariate logistic regression model, each 1 mmHg higher IOP SD was associated with 31% higher odds of developing progression. According to the study, eyes with an IOP SD < 3 mmHg remained stable over time, whereas eyes with an IOP SD ≥ 3 mmHg demonstrated significant progression. Several factors have been proposed to explain the different results with regards to the role of IOP fluctuation in the EMGT and the AGIS,[17] including different study designs, different populations and different outcome criteria. Although both studies calculated long-term IOP variation as the standard deviation of measurements over time, the AGIS calculations of IOP variation included measurements obtained after progression had occurred, whereas in the EMGT, measurements were obtained only up to the study endpoint. After progression occurred, it is possible that treatment would have been intensified and resulted in further IOP lowering and a consequent increase in IOP variation. This could have resulted in spurious positive relationship between IOP fluctuation and risk of progression in the AGIS investigation. In fact, when the EMGT data was re-analyzed including post-progression IOP measurements in the calculation of fluctuation, the authors also found IOP fluctuation to be related to progressive visual field damage.[21] A subsequently published reanalysis of the AGIS data by Caprioli and Coleman removing IOP data after progression found that IOP fluctuation was associated with risk of progression in patients with low, but not in those with high pressure.

In designing or evaluating studies of the relationship between IOP fluctuation and risk of glaucoma development and progression, it is important to recognize that variation is usually correlated with the level of mean IOP. Eyes with higher mean IOP tend to have higher variation. Therefore, when developing multivariate models to investigate the risk attributable to long-term IOP variation, it is important to adjust for mean IOP level.

4.1.2.2. Role of 24-hour IOP fluctuation as a risk factor for glaucoma

One prospective study assessed the relationship of same-day IOP fluctuations on risk of glaucoma progression.[23] Although this study suggested that IOP fluctuations are an independent risk factor for glaucoma, it used home tonometry to assess IOP fluctuations during the day, which can be a potentially unreliable method.[24] On the contrary, several retrospective studies have reported conflicting results.[25-28] Bergea *et al.*[26] studied the long-term effects of primary laser trabeculoplasty vs. pilocarpine eyedrops in 76 patients with newly diagnosed open-angle glaucoma. Patients were followed for up to 24 months. They obtained up to 12 diurnal IOP curves for each patient and evaluated the predictive value of six IOP parameters. They demonstrated improved preservation of visual fields in patients with smaller IOP fluctuations. However, they did not adjust for the confounding effects of follow-up mean IOP and follow-up IOP range simultaneously in the same model. Collaer *et al.*[25] reviewed the records of 93 consecutive glaucoma patients who underwent sequential office IOP measurements (every hour from 7 am to 5 pm on a single day). The authors found that 35% of progressing patients had an IOP range greater than 5 mmHg and concluded that the IOP range may be more important than IOP peak. Jonas *et al.*[28] studied the effect of 24-h IOP (five measurements) on glaucoma progression in a large group of patients with glaucoma and ocular hypertension. They suggested that it was the absolute IOP itself rather than its fluctuation that had the most significant effect on glaucoma progression. This study was limited by its design (registry study) and use of different antiglaucoma drugs with various IOP-lowering effects. Choi *et al.*[27] performed a retrospective chart review to evaluate the effect of 24-h IOP fluctuations in 113 patients with so-called 'normal-tension glaucoma'. Measurements were taken every two hours in a hospital setting. They found that both fluctuations in IOP and ocular perfusion pressure were related to worsening of glaucoma on both functional and structural tests. The strength of this study was the fact that patients had no previous or current use of antiglaucoma medications to confound the results.

Table 1 provides a summary of these studies. Differences in study design,

Table 1. Summary of studies evaluating the effect of IOP fluctuations as a risk factor for glaucoma for glaucoma development and progression.

Studies (year)	Design	Population	IOP measurement	Limitations
In support of IOP fluctuations as a risk factor				
CIGTS, 2011	Retrospective subset analysis; N = 578 participants	Newly detected glaucoma	Every 3 months until last visit	Retrospective; SD used as surrogate for fluctuation
AGIS, 2008	Retrospective subset analysis; N = 301 eyes	Advanced glaucoma	3 months after intervention; every 6 months thereafter	Retrospective; SD used as surrogate for fluctuation; Only IOPs after surgery and until evidence of progression used
Choi *et al.*, 2007[27]	Retrospective chart review; N = 113 eyes	POAG (NTG)	24-h IOP (every 2-3 hours)	Retrospective
Collaer *et al.*, 2005[25]	Retrospective chart review;N = 185 eyes	POAG	DTC (hourly 7 am to 5 pm)	Retrospective
Asrani *et al.*, 2000[23]	Prospective; N = 105 eyes	OAG	24-h IOP	Home monitoring by patients
Against IOP fluctuations as a risk factor				
DIGS, 2008	Subset analysis; N = 252 eyes	Untreated ocular hypertension	Annual	SD used as surrogate for fluctuation
EMGT, 2007	Retrospective subset analysis; N = 255 eyes	Newly detected untreated glaucoma	3 months after assignment to treatment to time of progression or last visit	Retrospective; SD used as surrogate for fluctuation
Malmö OHTS, 2005	Retrospective subset analysis; N = 90 eyes	Ocular hypertension	DTC (8 am, 11:30 am and 3:30 pm); every 3 months	Few IOP measurements during the day
Jonas *et al.*, 2007[28]	Registry study; N = 855 eyes	POAG	Minimum of 2 DTCs (5 pm, 9 pm, midnight, 7 am and noon)	Retrospective; Patients on different antiglaucoma medications
Bergea *et al.*, 1999[26]	Retrospective analysis; N = 82 eyes	Newly detected POAG	DTC (3 measurements) every 3 months	Retrospective

definitions, data analysis, and study populations may explain these apparently contradictory findings. Singh and Sit provided additional explanation for these discrepancies.[29] They suggested that the percentage of IOP variability would be a better measure of glaucoma risk than absolute change. Use of standard deviation of the mean IOP as a surrogate for variability (as in previously mentioned studies) captures only absolute changes and may underestimate the risk at low IOPs and overestimate the risk at higher IOPs.

It should be emphasized that the prognostic value of 24-h IOP fluctuations has never been evaluated in properly designed longitudinal studies. As described above, the few available studies are limited by the use of imperfect surrogates for the 24-h IOP variations.

4.2. Provocative Testing

The search for a clinically-useful provocative test in glaucoma, analogous to a cardiac stress test or glucose tolerance test, has been sought for many decades. Ideally, such a test would identify those individuals at highest risk of developing glaucoma or progressing. Both steroid and water-drinking tests were first introduced in the 1950s and 1960s. The steroid provocative test has proven to be of limited value in screening patients for glaucoma. The ability of IOP response to a topically-applied synthetic steroid to predict the development of glaucomatous visual field loss was not as good as the predictive power of a multivariate model that included patient age, race, baseline IOP, baseline outflow facility, baseline cup/disk ratio, and systemic hypertension. At the present time, steroid provocative testing has been abandoned. There is also insufficient evidence supporting the role of postural and Ibopamine tests, as providing independent contribution to assess risk of glaucoma development and progression.

The water-drinking test (WDT) is a stress test that indirectly assesses the outflow capacity and has been proposed as the test to estimate IOP peaks not identified during office hours, as well as the instability of the outflow system of the eye. Previous studies have shown significant correlations between IOP peaks observed during the WDT and those measured during office visits or on modified diurnal tension curves.[30-32] De Moraes *et al.*[30] reported results on 22 patients with newly-diagnosed glaucoma who were started on ocular hypotensive medication and had a WDT at the beginning of follow-up. Patients were then followed for eight visits during a follow-up period ranging from six to 12 months. The IOP peak during the WDT was compared to the IOP peak detected during longitudinal office visits. The two peaks were significantly correlated (Spearman's rho = 0.76; $P < 0.001$). The 95% confidence limits of agreement (office peak IOP – WDT peak IOP) ranged from -5.6 mmHg to 1.8 mmHg.[30]

The WDT has also been used to assess the effect of hypotensive drugs in glaucoma as well as to compare the effectiveness of surgical versus medical treatment in lowering IOP.[33-37] In a study enrolling patients with apparently well-controlled IOP during office visits, elevations of IOP after the WDT were significantly higher in those who were receiving medications compared to those who had undergone trabeculectomy (average increase of 40% versus 13%, respectively). This finding seems to suggest that the WDT may be able to uncover IOP peaks that are not detected during office visit. In fact, previous studies have suggested that WDT responses may be associated with glaucoma progression.[38-41] A study by Susanna and colleagues[38] followed 76 eyes of patients with open-angle glaucoma for an average of 26 months with an average of 4.6 visual field tests. Mean baseline MD of included eyes was approximately -9 dB. Twenty-eight (36.8%) of the eyes had visual field progression during follow-up according to the criteria used by the authors. The mean peak IOP detected during the WDT was 16.8 mmHg in progressing eyes versus 14.9 mmHg in non-progressing eyes, for a mean difference of 1.9 mmHg. Interestingly, among eyes that reached visual field progression, 25% showed IOP greater than 21 mmHg during the WDT versus only 4.2% in the stable group. Interestingly, a study published by Armaly and colleagues several decades ago also found that the response to the WDT was a risk factor for development of visual field defect in a large group of over 5,000 subjects of having the disease followed over time.[40]

Studies evaluating the reproducibility of the WDT have shown excellent reproducibility of the peak IOP during the test among treated and untreated glaucoma patients.[41,42] In patients who underwent the WDT at close intervals without changes in therapy, differences in IOP peaks during the WDT were within 2 mmHg in almost 90% of cases.

In summary, there is evidence that the WDT could potentially serve as a 'stress' test indirectly investigating the ability of the outflow system of the eye in handling pressure elevations.[35,38,44,45] Good correlation has been shown between peak IOP from the WDT and those acquired during office visits in the long-term. As the WDT can be performed quickly in the office, it could potentially serve as a surrogate measure indicative of IOP control. Further studies are necessary to clarify the additional benefit of the WDT over IOP measurements performed during clinic visits, *i.e.*, whether the peak IOP obtained during the WDT adds significant value in predicting clinically relevant outcomes in glaucoma in addition to (and not only compared to) longitudinal office-based IOP measurements. In addition, standardization of testing protocols in relation to volume of water necessary according to body weight, need for fasting, number and timing of IOP measurements, is necessary.

4.3. Ocular Perfusion Pressure

As described above, different clinical and epidemiological studies have demonstrated a strong correlation between the level of intraocular pressure and the prevalence and incidence of glaucomatous damage. Glaucoma occurs in eyes with 'normal' IOP (the range of IOP found in 95% of eyes without disease), but with increasing frequency as the IOP increases, without a clearly defined cut-off level below which the eye is safe and above which the eye is certain to be harmed. The occurrence of glaucomatous damage therefore seems to depend on the susceptibility of an individual optic nerve head (ONH) structure to a given level of IOP.[46,47] The existence of patients who develop glaucoma or have progressive disease despite low levels of IOP may suggest contributing pathogenic factors other than IOP. Abnormal ocular blood flow physiology and large variation of ocular perfusion pressure (IOP in relation to BP) are among the suggested risk factors for the damage to the ONH structure in glaucoma.[27,48-51]

Ocular perfusion pressure is the driving force for the blood circulation in the eye and is defined as the difference between the mean arterial blood pressure (MAP) and venous pressure. The venous pressure in the eye should be marginally higher than the intraocular pressure (IOP) for the vein to maintain an open lumen for blood circulation. Therefore, the perfusion pressure for intraocular vessels is often estimated as the mean ophthalmic arterial pressure (arbitrarily defined as 2/3 the brachial arterial pressure) minus the venous pressure, which is approximately the IOP. The mean ocular perfusion pressure (MOPP) is estimated from the mean brachial arterial pressure and IOP with the formula:[52]

$$MOPP = 2/3[DBP + 1/3\ (SBP - DBP)] - IOP$$

where DBP and SBP are the brachial diastolic and systolic blood pressures respectively.

IOP and BP and, therefore, MOPP have physiologic circadian variations, but the peaks and troughs in circadian IOP and BP do not necessarily occur simultaneously. In fact, there are times during the day such as early hours of morning during which high IOP coincides with relatively low BP and results in low ocular perfusion pressure.[51,53] In healthy individuals, the ocular blood flow is autoregulated through the change in the resistance of vessels to keep the tissue blood flow and metabolic activity stable, thus preserving the integrity of the tissue in the face of changes in MOPP.[52] It has been demonstrated that those with perfusion pressure lower than 50 mmHg are at a greater risk for OAG and at 30 mmHg the risk is four times greater.[54,55]

Several population-based studies have demonstrated the association between low perfusion pressure and risk of glaucoma. The results of the Baltimore Eye Survey indicated that lower perfusion pressure was strongly associated with an increased prevalence of POAG, and that POAG was associated with an alteration in factors related to ocular blood flow and a breakdown of autoregulation.[55] The Baltimore Eye Survey also found that systemic hypertension was protective in early glaucoma, possibly due to an increase in ocular perfusion pressure. However, late in hypertension, the risk of glaucoma was increased and it was suggested that vascular sclerosis reduced blood flow despite an elevated blood pressure.[56] The Barbados study[57] found that lower perfusion pressure at baseline increased the adjusted relative risk of OAG approximately three folds, and the Egna-Neumarkt Study[54] and the Proyecto VER[58] demonstrated that reduced diastolic perfusion pressure was an important risk factor for POAG.

It is important to emphasize that statistical analysis has difficulty determining whether OPP is an independent risk factor for glaucoma because intraocular pressure measurements are actually included in the formula used to calculate OPP. Therefore, unless an independent method is used to measure OPP, it is not possible currently to completely separate the effect of OPP from that of IOP.[59]

4.4. Corneal Thickness

4.4.1. How important is CCT as a risk factor?

Goldmann and Schmidt first discussed the influence of variations in corneal thickness and scleral rigidity on applanation tonometry.[60] Ehlers *et al.* reported that the Goldmann tonometer provided accurate readings only when the CCT was 0.52 mm; they calculated that applanation tonometry overestimated or underestimated IOP by approximately 5 mmHg for every 0.070 mm of deviation in corneal thickness.[61] Whitacre *et al.* reported that thin corneas may result in a 4- to

9-mmHg underestimation of IOP, and thick corneas may result in overestimation of the IOP by 6.8 mmHg.[62]

A large population based study of South Indian population by Vijaya *et al.* reported that a 100 µm increase in CCT was associated with a 1.96 mmHg increase in intraocular pressure in the rural population, and with 2.45 mmHg for every 100 µm in the urban population.[63]

In the Ocular Hypertension Treatment Study (OHTS), a low CCT value was identified as a risk factor for conversion of patients with ocular hypertension to POAG.[2] In OHTS, the authors divided the entire sample into three approximately equal-sized groups of thin (< 555 µm), intermediate (556-588 µm) and thick corneas (> 588 µm) and computed the multivariate hazard ratio for the development of POAG. Compared with participants with the thickest corneas, participants with intermediate central corneal measurements had a hazard ratio of 1.7, and participants with the thinnest central corneal measurements had a hazard ratio of 3.4.[2]

Findings from various reports suggest that the presence of a thin cornea is linked not only to the development of glaucoma among patients with OHT, but also to the severity of disease in OHT and POAG.[2,64-67] In OHT and OAG, a thin cornea was found out to be more strongly associated with disease severity than IOP.[2,67] Herndon *et al.* demonstrated that CCT was more strongly associated with the disease severity (mean deviation-MD on visual field and cup : disc-C:D ratio) as compared to IOP and age.[67] For every 10 µm increase in CCT, MD improved by 0.34 db and vertical C:D ratio decreased by 0.008.[67]

4.4.2. Is CCT a truly independent (not only statistically independent) risk factor for glaucoma development?

The Ocular Hypertension Treatment Study (OHTS) showed that central corneal thickness (CCT) was a significant predictor of which patients with ocular hypertension are at higher risk for converting to glaucoma. In a multivariable model including age, baseline intraocular pressure (measured by Goldmann tonometer), optic disc topography (cup/disc ratio) and visual field (pattern standard deviation), CCT retained its statistical significance as a predictor of glaucoma development, with a hazard ratio of 1.82 for each 40 µm thinner CCT. The results of this report have been mistakenly interpreted by some as demonstrating that CCT is an independent risk factor for the development of glaucoma. As Goldmann applanation tonometry (GAT) measurements ultimately depend on CCT, it is impossible in the original model to completely disentangle the effects of both. For example, consider two patients with the same baseline GAT IOP of 24 mmHg, but with corneal thicknesses of 520 μm and 560 μm. The adjusted hazard ratio for CCT in the OHTS multivariable model would tell us that the risk for developing glaucoma for the one with the thin cornea would be 82% higher. However, it is impossible to determine, from the original analysis, whether the increased risk is due to a true independent effect of corneal thickness *per se*, or simply due to the effect of CCT on GAT measurement error. In fact, using a correction formula proposed by Ehlers et al, the patient with the thinner cornea would have 'corrected' IOP close to the measured value of 24 mmHg. In contrast, the 'corrected' IOP would be 2.8 mmHg lower at approximately 21 mmHg for the patient with the thicker cornea. So, the increased risk could ultimately be due just to the fact that the first patient actually has a higher 'true' IOP. On the other hand, some authors have suggested that the predictive effect of CCT is not fully accounted for by its induced GAT measurement error, but rather that there is a possible association between corneal thickness and structural measures possibly related to glaucoma risk, such as scleral or lamina cribrosa thickness.

Lesk *et al.* investigated changes in optic nerve head topography and blood flow after therapeutic intraocular pressure reduction and correlated them with central corneal thickness.[68] Lamina cribrosa compliance was estimated using scanning confocal laser tomography by examining the position of the base of the cup relative to the retinal surface after intraocular pressure (IOP) changes. They suggested that patients with OHT and POAG with thin central corneas have greater forward displacement of the base of the cup, a surrogate marker for lamina cribrosa position, following IOP reduction than their cohorts with thicker central corneas. Patients with thin central corneas also seem to have smaller improvements in neuroretinal rim blood flow after IOP reduction than patients with thicker central corneas. These results suggest that a thin central cornea may be a marker for physiological differences in the biomechanical properties of the lamina cribrosa. In other words, it may be that a thin central cornea is connected to a thin sclera, which, in turn, is connected to a thin lamina.[68]

Brandt *et al.* attempted to shed light on this issue. They evaluated whether the OHTS prediction model could be improved by correcting IOP for CCT using previously published formulas. The rationale of the authors was that if the influence of CCT on GAT fully explains the role of CCT as a predictive factor, than inclusion of CCT-corrected IOP values in the model would cause CCT to become non-significant. They showed that models with CCT-corrected IOP did not perform better than the original model, as evaluated by c-statistics and calibration chi-squares. Additionally, CCT remained a statistically significant predictor in the multivariable model including CCT-corrected IOP. Based on these results, the authors concluded that the influence of corneal thickness as a prognostic factor for POAG is not entirely from its effect on IOP measurement error, but rather that CCT is a biomarker for structural and physical factors involved in the pathogenesis of glaucoma. However, a close analysis of the data actually suggested a decrease in the predictive ability of CCT when CCT-corrected IOP values were included in the model. The hazard ratios for CCT decreased from 1.84 in the original model to 1.38 in the model which included IOP corrected by the Ehlers formula, for example. More importantly, it is likely that correction formulas dot not fully capture the corneal-induced error on tonometric measurement. It has been shown that other factors besides corneal thickness may influence tonometric readings, such as corneal elasticity and viscoelasticity, and the correction formulas do not fully take into account these factors. The only way to fully evaluate the independent role of CCT as a prognostic factor would be to include in the predictive model IOP measurements obtained by a perfectly cornea-independent tonometer. In the reanalysis of OHTS data, the predictive abilities were similar between the original OHTS model including CCT and the models which did not include CCT, but only CCT-corrected IOP. This could actually imply that CCT is relatively unimportant for the final predictive ability of the multivariable model, as long as one includes CCT-corrected IOP.

The conclusion that CCT is a true independent risk factor for glaucoma is not validated at this time and requires further investigations.

4.4.3. Should IOP measurements be corrected by CCT?

Studies indicate that patients with NTG have a thinner CCT than do patients with POAG or normal individuals. Underestimation of the IOP in patients with POAG who have thin corneas may lead to a misdiagnosis of NTG, while overestimation of the IOP in normal subjects who have thick corneas may lead to a misdiagnosis of OHT.[69-71]

A few CCT-based correction formulae have been developed, however, their use in general is not recommended in clinical practice. In a masked, prospective clinical trial, Kohlhaas M *et al.*[72] examined 125 eyes of 125 patients scheduled for cataract surgery and cannulated the anterior chamber before surgery. Intraocular pressure (IOP) was set to 20, 35, and 50 mmHg in a closed system by means

thickness (CCT) does not necessarily help with decision making for an individual patient. If we can show, in an individual patient, that progression is occurring by robust structural or functional means, or both, then clearly the IOP needs to be lowered, regardless of the measurement performed and bias or error that may be included in that measurement.

To conclude, patients with POAG, OHT or NTG or glaucoma suspects should undergo ultrasound pachymetry at baseline examination for correct diagnosis. Thin CCT should be interpreted as a risk factor for development and progression for glaucoma. Consideration about more aggressive treatment and closer follow-up should be given to this patients. Repetition of CCT measurement on follow-ups is usually not recommended.

4.5. Corneal Hysteresis

Corneal hysteresis (CH) is a measure of the viscoelastic damping properties of the cornea, which can be estimated by analyzing the ability of the cornea to resist deformation induced by a pulse of air. CH may be evaluated *in vivo* using the Ocular Response Analyzer (ORA; Reichert Ophthalmic Instruments Inc, Depew, New York, USA), a device that delivers a metered air pulse to the cornea, while monitoring resulting changes in corneal curvature using a detector system.

Biomechanical studies in non-human primates with experimental glaucoma have shown that IOP elevation results in displacement of the lamina cribrosa and expansion of the scleral canal. These changes are thought to contribute to glaucomatous retinal ganglion cell loss as a result of mechanical pressure on retinal ganglion cell axons passing through the lamina pores. Hysteresis is a physical property related to the ability of connective tissues to dampen pressure changes. As the cornea and sclera are contiguous parts of the corneo-scleral envelope, formed from continuous extracellular matrix, deformability of the cornea and sclera are likely to be closely related. Thus, measures of CH could be indicative of susceptibility of the optic nerve head to IOP-induced biomechanical changes. High CH has been found in a clinical study of human eyes to be associated with greater posterior displacement of the optic nerve head on acute IOP elevation. In contrast, low CH as been associated with increased risk of glaucoma progression.[76-78] A possible explanation for these observations is that the optic nerve head of eyes with high CH may be more able to compensate for raised IOP. In contrast, the lamina and peripapillary sclera of eyes with lower CH would be less able to dampen IOP changes, potentially exposing retinal ganglion cells to greater mechanical strain with IOP elevation.

Several investigators have found an association between CH and optic nerve head morphology changes. Eyes with lower CH have been found to have larger cup-to-disc ratio and deeper cup, independently of IOP.[79] Cross-sectional studies have also shown that patients with glaucoma have lower CH values than healthy subjects and patients with bilateral asymmetric disease have lower CH in the eye with more severe damage.[80] Patients with lower CH are also at higher risk of progressive visual field loss[76-78] and progressive loss of the retinal nerve fiber layer.[81] In a prospective longitudinal study, Medeiros and colleagues[78] showed eyes with lower CH to have faster rates of visual field loss than those with higher CH; CH accounted for three times as much of progression as CCT in this study. This suggests that CH might be an important factor to consider in the assessment of the risk of progression in patients with glaucoma.

4.6. Myopia

A meta-analysis based on 11 population-based cross-sectional studies indicates that individuals with any myopia have approximately double the risk of developing open angle glaucoma in comparison with individuals without myopia. The pooled ORs were 2.46 (95%CI: 1.93-3.15) for high myopia (≤ -3D) and 1.77 (95%CI: 1.41-2.23) for low myopia (up to -3D).[82] Clinical case-control studies tend to report a higher OR but may be subject to selection bias.[83] A population-based longitudinal study reported an association between high myopia and incident OAG with an hazard ratio of 2.31 (95%CI: 1.19-4.49) but this association was not found in low myopia.[84]

Diagnosing glaucoma in the people with myopia, in particular high myopia, is challenging because they may share similar visual field changes and assessing cup-to-disc ratio and other glaucomatous disc change can be extremely difficult. This problem could lead to either under-diagnosis or over-diagnosis of glaucoma. Some methods based on imaging technologies such as OCT have been introduced to better differentiate glaucoma and myopia using the ganglion cell complex and its ratio to macular outer retinal thickness. As OAG produces progressive optic disc damage, glaucomatous progression is needed to confirm the diagnosis and therefore longitudinal observation from an established, well-defined baseline is important to achieve correct diagnosis.

Myopic eyes, and highly myopic especially, have a longer globe, thinner lamina cribosa and thinner scleral wall. They are perhaps more susceptible to

IOP elevation, structural collapse and having postoperative complications such as hypotony after filtration surgery. Post-LASIK eyes would create difficulties for IOP measurement and subsequent treatment.

4.7. Optic Disc Hemorrhages

Disc hemorrhage is rare in a healthy population (≤ 0.2%) and is a sign of glaucoma progression. In eyes of individuals suspected of having glaucoma, results from the Ocular Hypertension Treatment Study (OHTS) study suggested that the presence of disc hemorrhage would indicate a six times increased risk of developing glaucoma.[85]

4.8. Predictive Models (Risk Calculators)

Although the information on individual risk factors may already help clinicians in management decisions, it is frequently difficult to integrate the information on the several risk factors and provide a global assessment for a particular patient.[86] In that situation, predictive models or risk calculators may benefit clinicians in providing a more objective assessment of risk. Mansberger *et al.*[87] performed a survey of ophthalmologists to estimate their ability to predict the risk of glaucoma development in ocular hypertensive patients.[87] Ophthalmologists had the benefit of an oral review and written handouts summarizing the OHTS results. They found that ophthalmologists tended to underestimate the risk when compared to the actual risk found by a risk calculator. Ophthalmologists also had a large range of predictions, sometimes differing from the actual risk by 40%, illustrating the need for a more standardized method for risk assessment.

The development of predictive models (or risk calculators) involves use of statistical methods to develop models for prediction of outcome using one or more explanatory variables. Mansberger proposed the first calculator to estimate risk of developing glaucoma, based on analysis of the OHTS results.[88] Subsequently, Medeiros and colleagues published in 2005 the results on the development of the first validated risk calculator to assess the risk of an ocular hypertensive patient to develop glaucoma.[9] The risk calculator was derived based on the results published by the OHTS[2,89] and incorporated the variables that were described by that study as being significantly associated with the risk of developing glaucoma over time. The risk calculator was designed to estimate the chance of an ocular hypertensive patient to develop glaucoma if left untreated for five years. To simplify the use of the risk calculator, a point system and an electronic version of the calculator were made available for clinicians.

A predictive model that is derived from a particular dataset is not guaranteed to work on a different group of patients. In fact, the performance of regression models (or risk calculators) used as diagnostic or prediction tools is generally better on the dataset on which the model has been constructed (derivation set) compared to the performance of the same model on new data. Therefore, before risk calculators can be successfully incorporated into clinical practice they need to be validated on different populations. By validation we mean establishing that the risk calculator works satisfactorily for patients other than those from whose data the model was derived. Along with the steps involved in the development of the risk calculator, the results of its validation on an independent population of 126 patients with ocular hypertension were also presented.[9]

Several steps were taken to validate the OHTS-derived model. In the first step, the importance of the prognostic variables that had been previously identified by the OHTS study was evaluated on the new data set. All the variables had similar performance, except for diabetes mellitus, which was not significantly associated with the risk of developing glaucoma. Subsequently, the predictive performance of the model was investigated on the new data set. The ability of the OHTS-derived risk calculator to discriminate subjects who developed glaucoma from those who did not was reasonably good with a c-index of approximately 0.7. The c-index is a measure of the discriminating ability of a model (similar to the area under the Receiver Operating Characteristic [ROC] curve) and a c-index of 0.7 indicates that, in approximately 70% of the cases, the model allocated a higher predicted probability for a subject who actually developed glaucoma than for a subject who did not. The closer the c-index gets to 1, the better the discriminating ability of the model. The values of c-index found for the OHTS-derived risk calculator when applied to the independent cohort were similar to those found when risk models such as the Framingham coronary prediction scores are used to predict coronary heart disease events.[90,91] D'Agostino *et al.* reported c-indexes ranging from 0.63 to 0.83 when the Framingham functions were applied to six different cohorts of patients.[91]

The OHTS-derived risk calculator also had a good calibration when applied to the independent dataset. Checking calibration is another important step in validating a predictive model. A reliable or well-calibrated model will give predicted probabilities that agree numerically with the actual outcomes. For example, let us consider a group of 100 ocular hypertensive patients. If the model assigns an average probability of 12% for conversion to glaucoma for this group of subjects, it is expected that approximately 12 subjects will convert to glaucoma over time. That is, for a well-calibrated model, the predicted probabilities of conversion to glaucoma will agree closely with the observed probabilities of conversion. The OHTS-derived risk calculator performed well on the independent data set. For patients in whom the model predicted a high chance of converting to glaucoma, there was a high observed conversion rate; whereas for patients in whom the model predicted a low conversion rate, there was a low observed conversion rate.

In 2007, OHTS and EGPS investigators published results of the development and validation of a risk calculator for glaucoma based on the analysis of the combined OHTS/EGPS dataset.[8] The results were similar to the predictive model published in 2005, and the risk calculator contained the five variables significantly associated with the risk of glaucoma conversion: age, IOP, CCT, PSD and vertical cup/disc ratio. The risk model from the pooled OHTS/EGPS sample of over 1,100 ocular hypertension patients demonstrated excellent fit with a c-statistic of 0.74 and good calibration. The OHTS/EGPS risk calculator is available on the web at http://ohts.wustl.edu/risk.

4.8.1. Predictive models for glaucoma progression

Estimation of the risk of patients with existing glaucoma of developing progressive damage over time is at least as important as estimating the risk of unaffected patient developing glaucoma. The development of predictive models for glaucoma progression could use the same principles as those used to develop and validate models for glaucoma development. Initially, longitudinal studies that followed patients with glaucoma would have to be reviewed to identify risk factors associated with progressive disease.

Several studies have investigated the risk factors for progression in patients with established glaucomatous damage. The Early Manifest Glaucoma Trial (EMGT)[10] was designed specifically to evaluate the effect of IOP-lowering treatment on progression of glaucoma. The EMGT enrolled 255 newly diagnosed, previously untreated, open-angle glaucoma patients who had reproducible visual field defects at baseline. Patients with advanced visual field loss or IOP greater than 30 mmHg at baseline were excluded. Patients were randomized to 360° trabeculoplasty plus betaxolol versus no treatment. Eyes stayed in their allocation arms unless significant progression occurred. If the IOP in treated eyes exceeded 25 mmHg at two consecutive follow-ups or 35 mmHg in control eyes, latanoprost was added. Patients were followed for a median of six years, with excellent retention. Baseline IOP in treated and untreated groups were 20.6 ± 4.1 mmHg and 20.9 ± 4.1 mmHg, respectively. Mean IOP reduction was 25% in the treated group, with no changes in the control group. At study closure, the proportion of patients who developed progression was significantly larger in the control versus the treatment group (62% versus 45%, respectively; HR = 0.60; 95% CI: 0.42 – 0.84; P = 0.003). Differences between treated and untreated patients remained when results were stratified by baseline IOP level (< 21 mmHg or ≥ 21 mmHg), degree of visual field damage, age or presence of exfoliation.

Besides IOP, several other risk factors were identified by the EMGT as significantly associated with the risk of glaucoma progression: older age, exfoliation, presence of bilateral disease and worse mean deviation on the baseline visual fields. Recently, the EMGT also published results on the long-term follow-up of the original cohort and concluded that thinner central corneal thickness and decreased ocular perfusion pressure were also associated with higher risk of visual field progression over time.

A predictive model could theoretically be developed based on the results from the EMGT incorporating all the risk factors found to be significantly associated with progressive disease. Such a model would be helpful in estimating which glaucoma patients are at higher risk for developing progressive loss of visual function. It is important to emphasize that any predictive model developed on the basis of the EMGT or other studies evaluating risk factors for glaucoma progression would have to be validated on an independent population of patients, as described above for the risk calculators in ocular hypertension.

4.8.2. Limitations of predictive models

The use of predictive models in clinical practice has several limitations. Predictive models are based on restricted populations of patients that were selected based on strict inclusion and exclusion criteria and that may not be representative of all patients seen at everyday clinical settings. Use of these models should be restricted to those patients who are similar to the ones included in the studies used to develop and/or validate it. It is also important to emphasize that although predictive models can provide a more objective evaluation of risk, their use does not replace the judgment of a clinician when making management decisions. For example, current risk calculators to estimate risk of glaucoma development do not include important information to guide treatment such as medical health status and life expectancy, patient's willingness to treatment, costs of medications and overall effect of treatment on quality of life. Also, it is important to emphasize that current risk calculators for glaucoma have been designed to estimate the risk of development of the earliest signs of disease, which do not necessarily have an impact on the quality of vision of the patient. Finally, as more evidence regarding risk factors for disease development and progression accumulates, newer and better refined predictive models will be developed that should replace current existing ones.

References

1. Gordon MO, Kass MA. The Ocular Hypertension Treatment Study: design and baseline description of the participants. Arch Ophthalmol 1999;117(5):573-583.
2. Gordon MO, Beiser JA, Brandt JD, et al. The Ocular Hypertension Treatment Study: baseline factors that predict the onset of primary open-angle glaucoma. Arch Ophthalmol 2002;120(6):714-720; discussion 829-730.
3. Miglior S, et al. Results of the European Glaucoma Prevention Study. Ophthalmology 2005;112(3):366-375.
4. Miglior S, et al. The European glaucoma prevention study design and baseline description of the participants. Ophthalmology 2002;109(9):1612-1621.
5. Quigley HA. European Glaucoma Prevention Study. Ophthalmology 2005;112(9):1642-1643; author reply 1643-1645.
6. Parrish RK, 2nd. The European Glaucoma Prevention Study and the Ocular Hypertension Treatment Study: why do two studies have different results? Curr Opin Ophthalmol 2006;17(2):138-141.
7. European Glaucoma Prevention Study Group, et al. Predictive factors for open-angle glaucoma among patients with ocular hypertension in the European Glaucoma Prevention Study. Ophthalmology 2007;114(1):3-9.
8. Gordon MO, et al. Validated prediction model for the development of primary open-angle glaucoma in individuals with ocular hypertension. Ophthalmology 2007;114(1):10-19.
9. Medeiros FA, et al. Validation of a predictive model to estimate the risk of conversion from ocular hypertension to glaucoma. Arch Ophthalmol 2005;123(10):1351-1360.
10. Heijl A, et al. Reduction of intraocular pressure and glaucoma progression: results from the Early Manifest Glaucoma Trial. Arch Ophthalmol 2002;120(10):1268-1279.
11. Leske MC, et al. Factors for glaucoma progression and the effect of treatment: the early manifest glaucoma trial. Arch Ophthalmol 2003;121(1):48-56.
12. Collaborative Normal-Tension Glaucoma Study Group. Comparison of glaucomatous progression between untreated patients with normal-tension glaucoma and patients with therapeutically reduced intraocular pressures. Am J Ophthalmol 1998;126(4):487-497.
13. Anderson DR; Normal Tension Glaucoma Study Group. Collaborative normal tension glaucoma study. Curr Opin Ophthalmol 2003;14(2):86-90.
14. The AGIS Investigators. The Advanced Glaucoma Intervention Study (AGIS): The relationship between control of intraocular pressure and visual field deterioration. Am J Ophthalmol 2000;130(4):429-440.

15. Lichter PR, et al. Interim clinical outcomes in the Collaborative Initial Glaucoma Treatment Study comparing initial treatment randomized to medications or surgery. Ophthalmology 2001;108(11):1943-1953.
16. Lichter P, Musch DC, Gillespie BW, Niziol LN. Trabeculectomy as initial treatment for open-angle glaucoma patients with substantial visual field defects. Abstract presented at: American Glaucoma Society Annual Meeting, March 2006, Charleston, South Carolina.
17. Palmberg P. What is it about pressure that really matters in glaucoma? Ophthalmology 2007;114(2):203-204.
18. Miglior S, et al. Intercurrent factors associated with the development of open-angle glaucoma in the European Glaucoma Prevention Study. Am J Ophthalmol 2007;144(2):266-275.
19. Medeiros FA, Ng D, Zangwill L, Sample PA, Weinreb RN. Long-term intraocular pressure fluctuations and risk of conversion from ocular hypertension to glaucoma. ARVO abstract 2007.
20. Bengtsson B, Heijl A. Diurnal IOP fluctuation: not an independent risk factor for glaucomatous visual field loss in high-risk ocular hypertension. Graefes Arch Clin Exp Ophthalmol 2005;243(6):513-518.
21. Bengtsson B, Leske MC, Hyman L, Heijl A. Fluctuation of intraocular pressure and glaucoma progression in the early manifest glaucoma trial. Ophthalmology 2007;114(2):205-209.
22. Nouri-Mahdavi K, et al. Predictive factors for glaucomatous visual field progression in the Advanced Glaucoma Intervention Study. Ophthalmology 2004;111(9):1627-1635.
23. Asrani S, et al. Large diurnal fluctuations in intraocular pressure are an independent risk factor in patients with glaucoma. J Glaucoma 2000;9(2):134-142.
24. Tarkkanen A, Ulfves K, Ulfves T. Self-tonometry in glaucoma. Graefes Arch Clin Exp Ophthalmol 2010;248(11):1679-1681.
25. Collaer N, Zeyen T, Caprioli J. Sequential office pressure measurements in the management of glaucoma. J Glaucoma 2005;14(3):196-200.
26. Bergea B, Bodin L, Svedbergh B. Impact of intraocular pressure regulation on visual fields in open-angle glaucoma. Ophthalmology 1999;106(5):997-1004; discussion 1004-1005.
27. Choi J, et al. Circadian fluctuation of mean ocular perfusion pressure is a consistent risk factor for normal-tension glaucoma. Invest Ophthalmol Vis Sci 2007;48(1):104-111.
28. Jonas JB, Budde WM, Stroux A, Oberacher-Velten IM, Junemann A. Diurnal intraocular pressure profiles and progression of chronic open-angle glaucoma. Eye (Lond) 2007;21(7):948-951.
29. Singh K, Sit AJ. Intraocular pressure variability and glaucoma risk: complex and controversial. Arch Ophthalmol 2011;129(8):1080-10doi: 10.1001/archophthalmol.2011.Epub 2011 Apr
30. De Moraes CG, Furlanetto RL, Reis AS, et al. Agreement between stress intraocular pressure and long-term intraocular pressure measurements in primary open-angle glaucoma. Clin Experiment Ophthalmol 2009;37:270-274.
31. De Moraes CG, Susanna R Jr. Correlation between the water drinking test and modified diurnal tension curve in untreated glaucomatous eyes. Clinics 2008;63:433-436.
32. Kumar RS, de Guzman MH, Ong PY, et al. Does peak intraocular pressure measured by water-drinking test reflect peak circadian levels? A pilot study. Clin Experiment Ophthalmol 2008;36:312-315.
33. Susanna R Jr, Sheu WP. Latin American Glaucoma Society. Comparison of latanoprost with fixed-combination dorzolamide and timolol in adult patients with elevated intraocular pressure: an eight-week, randomized, open-label, parallel-group, multicenter study in Latin America. Clin Ther 2004;26:755-768.

34. Facio AC, Reis AS, Vidal KS, et al. A comparison of bimatoprost 0.03% versus the fixed-combination of latanoprost 0.005% and timolol 0.5% in adult patients with elevated intraocular pressure: an eight-week, randomized, open-label trial. J Ocul Pharmacol Ther 2009;25:447-451.
35. Medeiros FA, Pinheiro A, Moura FC, et al. Intraocular pressure fluctuations in medical versus surgically treated glaucomatous patients. J Ocul Pharmacol Ther 2002;18:489-498.
36. Guedes RA, Guedes VM, Chaoubah A. Use of water drinking test after non-penetrating deep sclerectomy. J Fr Ophtalmol 2005;28:1076-1080.
37. Germano RA, Susanna R Jr, De Moraes CG, et al. Effect of Switching From Latanoprost to Bimatoprost in Primary Open-Angle Glaucoma Patients Who Experienced Intraocular Pressure Elevation During Treatment. J Glaucoma 2016;25(4):359-366.
38. Susanna R Jr, Vessani RM, Sakata L, et al. The relation between intraocular pressure peak in the water drinking test and visual field progression in glaucoma. Br J Ophthalmol 2005;89:1298-1301.
39. Yoshikawa K, Inoue T, Inoue Y. Normal tension glaucoma: the value of predictive tests. Acta Ophthalmol 1993;71:463-470.
40. Armaly MF, Krueger DE, Maunder L, et al. Biostatistical analysis of the Collaborative Glaucoma Study I. Summary report of the risk factors for glaucomatous visual-field defects. Arch Ophthalmol 1980;98:2163-2171.
41. Susanna R, Jr., Hatanaka M, Vessani RM, et al. Correlation of asymmetric glaucomatous visual field damage and water-drinking test response. Invest Ophthalmol Vis Sci 2006;47(2):641-6
42. Babic M, De Moraes CG, Hatanaka M, et al. Reproducibility of the water drinking test in treated glaucomatous patients. Clin Experiment Ophthalmol 2015;43(3):228-2
43. Hatanaka M, Alencar LM, De Moraes CG, et al. Reproducibility of intraocular pressure peak and fluctuation of the water drinking test. Clin Experiment Ophthalmol 2013;41:355-359.
44. Kasim B. Muz E, Irkec M, Orhan M, Karabulut. Mikropoulos DG, Konstas AG. Intraocular Pressure Characteristics of Exfoliative Glaucoma and Mocan MC1 E. Exfoliation Syndrome as Determined With the Water Drinking Test. J Glaucoma 2016;25(3):301-305.
45. Landers J. Challenging glaucoma with the water-drinking test. Clin Exper Ophthalmol 2015;203:200-201.
46. Morrison JC, Johnson EC, Cepurna W, Jia L. Understanding mechanisms of pressure-induced optic nerve damage. Prog Retin Eye Res 2005;24(2):217-240.
47. Burgoyne CF, Downs JC, Bellezza AJ, Suh JK, Hart RT. The optic nerve head as a biomechanical structure: a new paradigm for understanding the role of IOP-related stress and strain in the pathophysiology of glaucomatous optic nerve head damage. Prog Retin Eye Res 2005;24(1):39-73.
48. Anderson DR, Drance SM, Schulzer M. Factors that predict the benefit of lowering intraocular pressure in normal tension glaucoma. Am J Ophthalmol 2003;136(5):820-829.
49. Cioffi GA, Alm A. Measurement of ocular blood flow. J Glaucoma 2001;10(5 Suppl 1):S62-64.
50. Flammer J, et al. The impact of ocular blood flow in glaucoma. Progress in retinal and eye research 2002;21(4):359-393.
51. Sehi M, Flanagan JG, Zeng L, Cook RJ, Trope GE. Relative change in diurnal mean ocular perfusion pressure: a risk factor for the diagnosis of primary open-angle glaucoma. Invest Ophthalmol Vis Sci 2005;46(2):561-567.
52. Gherghel D, Orgul S, Gugleta K, Gekkieva M, Flammer J. Relationship between ocular perfusion pressure and retrobulbar blood flow in patients with glaucoma with progressive damage. Am J Ophthalmol 2000;130(5):597-605.

53. Liu JH, Gokhale PA, Loving RT, Kripke DF, Weinreb RN. Laboratory assessment of diurnal and nocturnal ocular perfusion pressures in humans. Journal of ocular pharmacology and therapeutics : the official journal of the Association for Ocular Pharmacology and Therapeutics 2003;19(4):291-297.
54. Bonomi L, et al. Vascular risk factors for primary open angle glaucoma: the Egna-Neumarkt Study. Ophthalmology 2000;107(7):1287-1293.
55. Tielsch JM, Katz J, Sommer A, Quigley HA, Javitt JC. Hypertension, perfusion pressure, and primary open-angle glaucoma. A population-based assessment. Arch Ophthalmol 1995;113(2):216-221.
56. Sommer A. Glaucoma risk factors observed in the Baltimore Eye Survey. Curr Opin Ophthalmol 1996;7(2):93-98.
57. Leske MC, Wu SY, Nemesure B, Hennis A. Incident open-angle glaucoma and blood pressure. Arch Ophthalmol 2002;120(7):954-959.
58. Quigley HA, et al. The prevalence of glaucoma in a population-based study of Hispanic subjects: Proyecto VER. Arch Ophthalmol 2001;119(12):1819-1826.
59. Khawaja AP, Crabb DP, Jansonius NM. The role of ocular perfusion pressure in glaucoma cannot be studied with multivariable regression analysis applied to surrogates. Invest Ophthalmol Vis Sci 2013;54(7):4619-4620.
60. Goldmann H, Schmidt T. Uber Applanations tonometrie. Ophthalmologica 1957;134:221-242.
61. Ehlers N, Bramsen T, Sperling S. Applanation tonometry and central corneal thickness. Acta Ophthalmol (Copenh) 1975;53:34-43.
62. Whitacre MM, Stein RA, Hassanein K. The effect of corneal thickness on applanation tonometry. Am J Ophthalmol 1993;115:592-596.
63. Vijaya L, George R, Arvind H, et al. Central corneal thickness in adult South Indians: the Chennai Glaucoma Study. Ophthalmology 2010;117(4):700-704.
64. Medeiros FA, Sample PA, Weinreb RN. Corneal thickness measurements and frequency doubling technology perimetry abnormalities in ocular hypertensive eyes. Ophthalmology 2003;110:1903-1908.
65. Medeiros FA, Sample PA, Weinreb RN. Corneal thickness measurements and visual function abnormalities in ocular hypertensive patients. Am J Ophthalmol 2003;135:131- 137.
66. Medeiros FA, Sample PA, Zangwill LM, et al. Corneal thickness as a risk factor for visual field loss in patients with preperimetric glaucomatous optic neuropathy. Am J Ophthalmol 2003;136:805-813.
67. Herndon LW, Weizer JS, Stinnett SS. Central corneal thickness as a risk factor for advanced glaucoma damage. Arch Ophthalmol 2004;122:17-21.
68. Lesk MR, Hafez AL, Descovich D. Relationship between central corneal thickness and changes of optic nerve head topography and blood flow after intraocular pressure reduction in open-angle glaucoma and ocular hypertension. Arch Ophthalmol 2006;124(11):1568-1572.
69. Copt RP, Thomas R, Mermoud A. Corneal thickness in ocular hypertension, primary open-angle glaucoma, and normal tension glaucoma. Arch Ophthalmol 1999;117(1):14-16.
70. Ventura AC, Böhnke M, Mojon DS. Central corneal thickness measurements in patients with normal tension glaucoma, primary open angle glaucoma, pseudoexfoliation glaucoma, or ocular hypertension. Br J Ophthalmol 2001;85(7):792-795.
71. Shetgar AC, Mulimani MB. The central corneal thickness in normal tension glaucoma, primary open angle glaucoma and ocular hypertension. J Clin Diagn Res 2013;7(6):1063-1067.
72. Kohlhaas M, Boehm AG, Spoerl E, et al. Effect of central corneal thickness, corneal curvature,

and axial length on applanation tonometry. Arch Ophthalmol 2006;124(4):471-476.

73. Park SJ, Ang GS, Nicholas S, et al. The effect of thin, thick, and normal corneas on Goldmann intraocular pressure measurements and correction formulae in individual eyes. Ophthalmology 2012;119(3):443-449.
74. Umurhan Akkan JC, Akkan F, Sezgin Akcay BI, et al. Dynamic Contour Tonometry and Goldmann Applanation Tonometry: Difference of Intraocular Pressure Values Between Eyes with and without Glaucomatous Damage in Thin Corneas. Klin Monatsbl Augenheilkd 2015;232(10):1190-1197.
75. Doughty MJ, Zaman ML. Human corneal thickness and its impact on intraocular pressure measures: a review and meta-analysis approach. Surv Ophthalmol 2000;44(5):367-408.
76. Congdon NG, Broman AT, Bandeen-Roche K, Grover D, Quigley HA. Central corneal thickness and corneal hysteresis associated with glaucoma damage. Am J Ophthalmol 2006;141(5):868-875.
77. De Moraes CV, Hill V, Tello C, Liebmann JM, Ritch R. Lower corneal hysteresis is associated with more rapid glaucomatous visual field progression. J Glaucoma 2012;21(4):209-213.
78. Medeiros FA, et al. Corneal hysteresis as a risk factor for glaucoma progression: a prospective longitudinal study. Ophthalmology 2013;120(8):1533-1540.
79. Prata TS, et al. Association between corneal biomechanical properties and optic nerve head morphology in newly diagnosed glaucoma patients. Clin Exp Ophthalmol 2012;40(7):682-688.
80. Anand A, et al. Corneal hysteresis and visual field asymmetry in open angle glaucoma. Invest Ophthalmol Vis Sci 2010;51(12):6514-6518.
81. Zhang C, et al. Corneal Hysteresis and Progressive Retinal Nerve Fiber Layer Loss in Glaucoma. Am J Ophthalmol 2016;166:29-36.
82. Marcus MW, de Vries MM, Junoy Montolio FG, Jansonius NM. Myopia as a risk factor for open-angle glaucoma: a systematic review and meta-analysis. Ophthalmology 2011;118(10):1989-1994 e2.
83. Ponte F, Giuffré G, Giammanco R, Dardanoni G. Risk factors of ocular hypertension and glaucoma: the Casteldaccia Eye Study. Doc Ophthalmol 1994;85:203-210.
84. Czudowska MA, Ramdas WD, Wolfs RC, et al. Incidence of glaucomatous visual field loss: a ten-year follow-up from the Rotterdam Study. Ophthalmology 2010;117:1705-1712.
85. Budenz DL, et al. Detection and prognostic significance of optic disc hemorrhages during the Ocular Hypertension Treatment Study. Ophthalmology 2006;113(12):2137-2143.
86. Mansberger SL, Medeiros FA, Gordon M. Diagnostic tools for calculation of glaucoma risk. Surv Ophthalmol 2008;53 Suppl1:S11-16.
87. Mansberger SL, Cioffi GA. The probability of glaucoma from ocular hypertension determined by ophthalmologists in comparison to a risk calculator. J Glaucoma 2006;15(5):426-431.
88. Mansberger SL. A risk calculator to determine the probability of glaucoma. J Glaucoma 2004;13(4):345-347.
89. Coleman AL, Gordon MO, Beiser JA, Kass MA. Baseline risk factors for the development of primary open-angle glaucoma in the Ocular Hypertension Treatment Study. Am J Ophthalmol 2004;138(4):684-685.
90. Liu J, et al. Predictive value for the Chinese population of the Framingham CHD risk assessment tool compared with the Chinese Multi-Provincial Cohort Study. Jama 2004;291(21):2591-2599.
91. D'Agostino RB Sr, Grundy S, Sullivan LM, Wilson P. Validation of the Framingham coronary heart disease prediction scores: results of a multiple ethnic groups investigation. Jama 2001;286(2):180-187.

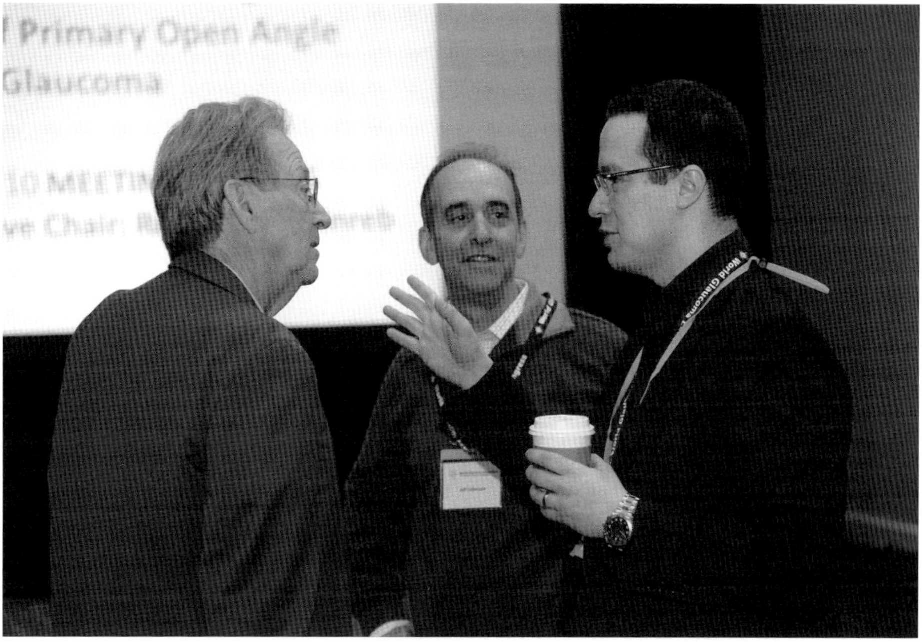

Don Hood, Jeff Liebmann and Gustavo De Moraes

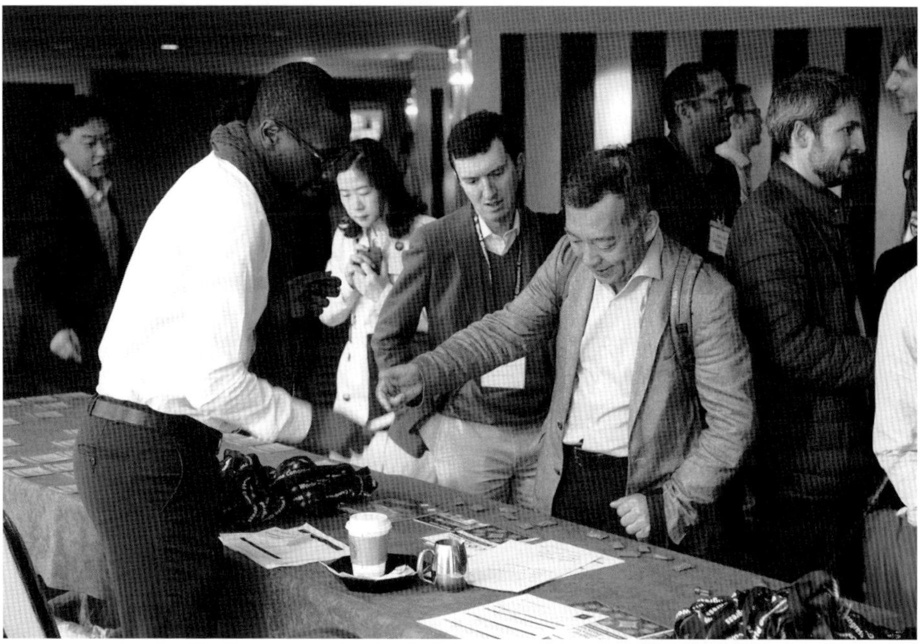

Makoto Aihara

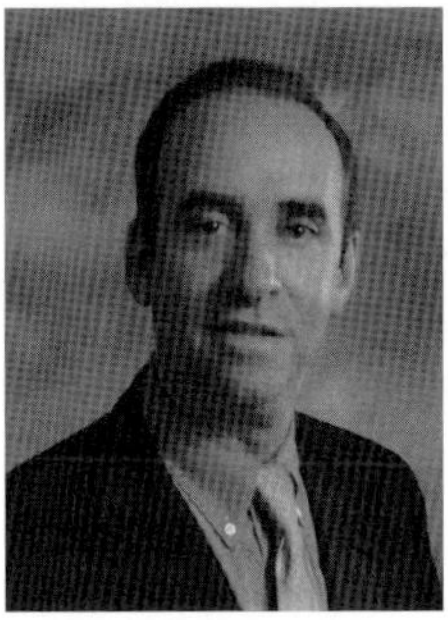

Jeffrey Liebmann

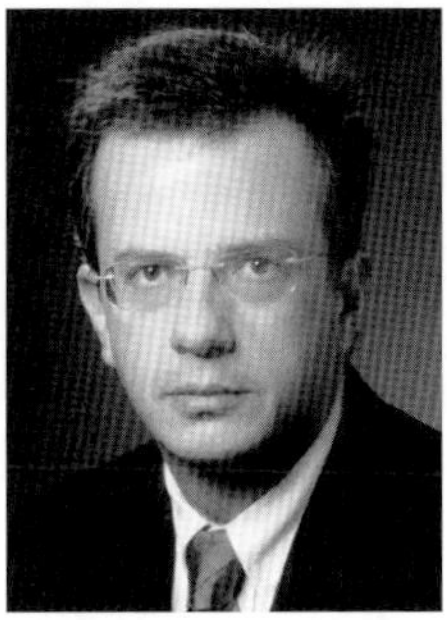

Fotis Topouzis

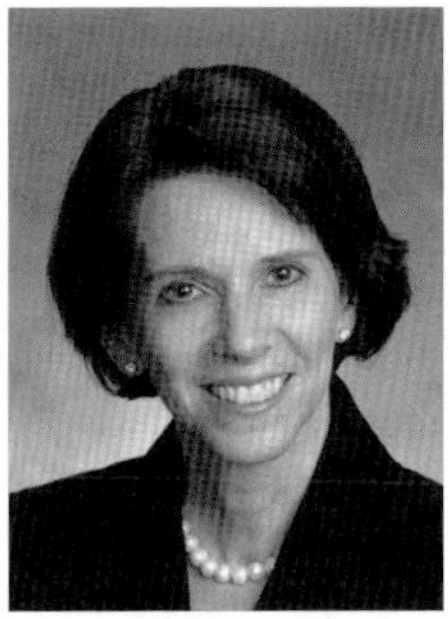

Janey Wiggs

5. RISK ASSESSMENT: SYSTEMIC FACTORS

Section leaders: Jeffrey Liebmann
Section co-leaders: Fotis Topouzis, Janey Wiggs
Contributors: Florent Aptel, Tin Aung, Rupert Bourne, Subhabrata Chakrabarti, Jonathan Crowston, Panayiota Founti, Neeru Gupta, Alon Harris, Jost Jonas, Kenji Kashiwagi, Michael Kook, Fabian Lerner, Kaweh Mansouri, Keith Martin, Sameh Mosaed, Jonathan Myers, Lou R. Pasquale, Bruce Prum, Robert Ritch, Leopold Schmetterer, Arthur Sit, Ingeborg Stalmans, Roy Wilson

Consensus statements

1. Primary open-angle glaucoma (POAG) occurs at all ages, and the incidence and prevalence accelerates with age.
2. Populations with the highest incidence and prevalence of POAG have African ancestry.
   Comment: Due to the earlier age of disease onset, the average duration of POAG may be greatest in individuals of African ancestry.
3. Hispanics may have higher incidence and prevalence of POAG than individuals of European ancestry (non-Hispanic whites).
4. Older age is a risk factor for glaucoma onset and progression.
5. Although an increased prevalence of POAG in men has been reported, there is not enough evidence to support an association of POAG risk with male gender.
6. Lower socioeconomic status may be associated with later presentation of POAG.
7. First-degree relatives of POAG patients are at higher risk for glaucoma.
8. Although genetic association studies have revealed multiple associated loci for POAG, there is little value for routine genetic testing to diagnose or predict the development of glaucoma at the current time.
9. There is consistent, but weak, positive association between diastolic blood

Diagnosis of Primary Open Angle Glaucoma, pp 161-187
Edited by Robert N. Weinreb, David Garway-Heath, Christopher Leung, Felipe Medeiros, Jeffrey Liebmann

5.1.1.2. Gender

Gender has been inconsistently associated with OAG prevalence, yet two meta-analyses of population-based glaucoma studies have reported higher prevalence of POAG in men than in women, Tham *et al.* reporting an OR of 1.36 (OR, 1.36; 95% CI, 1.23-1.52) after adjusting for age, habitation type, response rate, and year of study conducted,[17] and Rudnicka *et al.* reporting an OR of 1.37 (95% CI, 1.22-1.53).[27] Incidence of glaucoma was reported by the Barbados Eye Study to be higher in men than women (2.7% vs 1.9%).20 By combining population-based datasets, a study by Broman *et al.* reported no significant difference in progression rates between men and women.[22]

5.1.1.3. Race/ethnicity

A recent meta-analysis of 53 population-based glaucoma studies demonstrated the variation in prevalence of glaucoma across geographic regions and ethnic groups.[17] In those aged 40-80 years people of African ancestry had the highest prevalence of glaucoma (6.11%; 95% CI, 3.83-9.13) and POAG (5.40%; 95% CI, 3.17-8.27), while Asians had the highest prevalence of primary angle-closure glaucoma (PACG) (1.20%; 95% CI, 0.46-2.55).

As mentioned previously, the probability of incident POAG rises with age in all ethnicities in a greater than linear fashion, with the highest incidence in African--derived persons but differences by ethnicity narrow in older age groups.[22] In the same study using cross-sectional data, average duration of glaucoma since age of onset of POAG was shown to vary between ethnic groups, highest for African derived populations (15.4 years; 95% CI: 14.6-15.9), similar durations for European and Hispanic populations (13.1 years; 95% CI, 12.2-13.8 years and 13.0 years; 95% CI, 12.1-13.6 years, respectively) and shortest duration in Chinese (10.5 years; 95% CI, 8.8-12.6 years). The longer average duration of disease in African-derived persons is an important factor driving the greater progression and morbidity of POAG in this racial group. Broman *et al.* demonstrated that despite having a shorter life expectancy, African-derived persons have OAG for up to 2.3 years longer than European-derived persons.[22] This is a result of higher incidence of disease at an earlier age and probably other factors such as differential access to care and acceptance of and response to treatment. Average individual progression rate in the worse eye was not significantly different among the four ethnic groups but was numerically lowest among European-derived persons (1.12

dB/y) and highest among Chinese persons (1.56 dB/y). These progression rates calculated from population-based data are more rapid than those reported in clinic-based studies such as clinical trials (*e.g.*, Early Manifest Glaucoma Trial where untreated subjects showed a progression rate in MD of 0.6-0.8 dB/year[28]).

The unilateral blindness rate due to POAG has been reported as highest in African-derived and Chinese persons, compared with European and Hispanics.[22] In the OHTS study, African-Americans had a higher incidence of POAG measured as the cumulative proportion of ocular hypertensives converting to POAG at 13 years.[29] This racial difference was no longer significant when accounting for the larger baseline cup/disc ratios and thinner central corneas of this racial group in the analysis.

5.1.1.4. Socioeconomic status

The detection of POAG in most societies is a result of opportunistic case detection and therefore detection of early to moderate cases of asymptomatic glaucoma is reliant on ocular examinations of sufficient regularity and quality. Socioeconomic status has been shown to be positively correlated with knowledge of glaucoma and its treatment and in a Dutch study, the lowest socioeconomic group required a greater need for information on public assistance and practical aspects of glaucoma and more often expected that glaucoma damage could be repaired.[30] Lack of awareness was a major risk for late presentation in an Australian study, rather than the lack of access to care.[31] Additionally, socioeconomic status may affect eye care service utilization and healthcare seeking behavior and therefore the chance to identify asymptomatic glaucoma.[32] A recent study involving a nationwide healthcare database in Taiwan found that subjects who lived in urban areas or had more healthcare utilization were more likely to be diagnosed with glaucoma. Socioeconomic status in this study affected the diagnosis of POAG and PACG in different ways; subjects with lower socioeconomic status were more likely to be diagnosed as PACG, while those with higher socioeconomic status were more likely to be diagnosed as POAG.[33] Other population-based studies have cited lack of eye care visits as the major risk factor for undiagnosed POAG.[34,35] Subjects with higher socioeconomic status may more frequently access eye care because of regular preventive eye care visits or increased prevalence of myopia and associated retinopathy necessitating glasses prescription and fundus examination, whereupon glaucoma may be detected. Meta-analyses of population-based studies have detected increased prevalence of POAG in urban areas, which may be related to a higher prevalence of myopia, or alternatively easier and more access to healthcare in urban settings.[17]

Although some studies have suggested no link between deprivation and severity of glaucoma at presentation,[36] several hospital-based studies have reported low socioeconomic status to be a risk factor for advanced glaucoma at presentation.[37-39] It is unclear whether the advanced disease at diagnosis in subjects with low socio-economic status is the result of delayed diagnosis due to reduced accessibility and use of eye care facility or increased susceptibility.

5.1.1.5. Genetics

5.1.1.5.1. Genetic risk factors for POAG

Familial linkage studies have implicated chromosomal regions and genes showing significant linkage with POAG (such as Myocilin) and congenital glaucoma (such as CYP1B1). These genes show Mendelian inheritance with very strong disease penetrance, as opposed to the associated loci seen for sporadic glaucoma.

To date, genetic association studies have revealed multiple robustly associated loci for sporadic POAG. The spectrum of POAG loci are unexpectedly broad, implicating genes such as CDKN2B-AS for predominantly normal pressure glaucoma, CAV1-CAV2, TMCO1, and ABCA1 for high pressure glaucoma, as well as more recent findings such as AFAP1, GAS7, TXNRD2, and ATXN2 for POAG. GWAS studies have also identified genes associated with quantitative traits associated with POAG, such intraocular pressure (IOP), central cornea thickness and optic disc size. Unexpectedly, the number of genetic loci shared between the IOP and POAG phenotype is limited (CAV1-CAV2, TMCO1, ABCA1, and GAS7), suggesting that POAG susceptibility is not solely underlined by increases in IOP alone.

From a genetic perspective, POAG is also associated with some systemic diseases with strong Mendelian inheritance such as Marfan syndrome and osteo-genesis imperfect.

Moving forward, it is likely that the disease allelic spectrum could overlap between the familial (earlier onset) and sporadic forms (later onset) of glaucoma. The successful description of such an overlap will extend our understanding on disease biology and pathogenesis for glaucoma and could unveil potential therapeutic targets.

Table 1. POAG genetic loci identified from genome wide association studies (GWAS).

Gene	Index SNP	Effect allele	Odds Ratio (OR, p value)	Reference
CAV1/2	rs4236601	A	OR =1.36, Pmeta= 5.00×10^{-10}	Thorleiffson *et al.*, 2010[40]
CDKN2B-AS1	rs4977756	A	OR = 1.39, Pmeta= $4.7 \times 10^{--14}$	Burdon *et al.*, 2011[41]
SIX1/SIX6	rs10483727	A	OR = 1.32, Pmeta = 3.87×10^{-11}	Wiggs *et al.*, 2012[42]
TMCO1	rs4656461	G	OR = 1.68, Pmeta = 6.1×10^{-10}	Burdon *et al.*, 2011[41]
8q22	rs284489	G	OR=0.62 Pmeta =8.88×10^{-10}	Wiggs *et al.*, 2012[42]
ABCA1	rs2472493	G	OR = 1.31, Pmeta = 2.10×10^{-19}	Gharakani *et al.*, 2014[43]
AFAP1	rs4619890	G	OR = 1.20, Pmeta = 7.0×10^{-10}	Gharakani *et al.*, 2014[43]
GAS7	rs9913991	A	OR = 2.23 , Pmeta =9.8×10^{-9}	Hysi *et al.*, 2014[44]
GMDS	rs11969985	G	OR = 1.31, Pmeta = 7.7×10^{-10}	Gharakani *et al.*, 2014[43]
PMM2	rs3785176	G	OR = 1.31, Pmeta = 3.18×10^{-6}	Chen *et al.*, 2014[45]
TGFBR3-CDC7	rs1192415	G	OR =1.13, Pmeta = 1.60×10^{-8}	Li *et al.*, 2015[46]
TXNRD2	rs35934224	T	OR = 0.78, Pmeta = 4.05×10^{-11}	Bailey *et al.*, 2016[47]
ATXN2	rs7137828	T	OR = 1.17, Pmeta = 8.73×10^{-10}	Bailey *et al.*, 2016[47]
FOXC1	rs2745572	A	OR = 1.17, Pmeta = 1.76×10^{-10}	Bailey *et al.*, 2016[47]

Table 2. POAG Loci/genes identified from familial linkage analysis studies.

Locus	Region	Trait	Population	Identified POAG genes	Reference
GLC1A	1q21-q24	POAG	Multiple	MYOC	Stone *et al*., 1997[48]
GLC1B	2cen-q13	POAG	Caucasian	None	Stoilova *et al*., 1996[49]
GLC1C	3q21-q24	POAG	American	None	Wirtz *et al*., 1997[50]
GLC1D	8q23	POAG	American	None	Trifan *et al*., 1998[51]
GLC1E	10p14-p15	POAG	Multiple	OPTN	Rezaie *et al*., 2002[52]
GLC1F	7q35-q36	POAG	American	ASB10	Pasutto *et al*., 2012[53]
GLC1G	5q22.1	POAG	Multiple	WDR36	Monemi *et al*., 2005[54]
GLC1H	2p15-p16	POAG	Caucasian	None	Suriyapperuma *et al*., 2007[55]
GLC1I	15q11-q13	POAG	American	None	Woodroffe *et al*., 2006[56]
GLC1J	9q22	POAG	American	None	Wiggs *et al*., 2004[57]
GLC1K	20p12	POAG	American	None	Wiggs *et al*., 2004[57]
GLC1L	3p21-22	POAG	Australian	None	Sherwin *et al*., 2009[58]
GLC1M	5q22.1-q32	JOAG	Chinese	None	Fan *et al*., 2007[59]
GLC1N	15q22-24	JOAG	Chinese	None	Aragon-Martin *et al*., 2008[60]
GLC1O	19q13	POAG	Caucasian, Asian	NTF4	Pasutto *et al*., 2009[61]
GLC1P	12q14	NTG/CODA	American	None	Fingert *et al*., 2011[62]
GLC1Q	4q35.1-q35.2	POAG	Caucasian	None	Porter *et al*., 2011[63]

Table 3. Primary congenital glaucoma loci/genes identified from familial linkage analysis studies.

Locus	Region	Trait	Population	Identified genes	Reference
GLC3A	2p21	PCG	Multiple	**CYP1B1**	Stoilov *et al.*, 1997[64]
GLC3B	1p36	PCG	Turkish	None	Akarsu *et al.*, 1996[65]
GLC3C	14q24	PCG	Multiple	**LTBP2**	Narooie-Nejad *et al.*, 2009[66]

5.1.2. Cardiovascular system

Louis Pasquale, Florent Aptel, Alon Harris, Panayiota Founti, Michael Kook, Ingeborg Stalmans

5.1.2.1. Systolic and diastolic blood pressure

A. Hypertension

Overall, the relation between systemic hypertension (HTN) and primary open-angle glaucoma (POAG) varies from null to adverse as described in two meta-analytical papers that provide a comprehensive overview of worked published up to 2012.[67,68] One study not captured in these meta-analytical works actually found an inverse relation between (HTN) and open-angle glaucoma (OAG).[69] Collectively the papers that constitute these meta-analyses vary considerably in terms of how IOP and BP were measured, how HTN and POAG were defined, study design and covariate adjustment. Nonetheless, there is robust evidence for a positive association between increases in systolic BP and increases in IOP and between increases in diastolic BP and IOP – these associations are consistent across both cross-sectional and longitudinal studies. Overall, a 10 mmHg increase in systolic BP was associated with a 0.26 mmHg increase in IOP and a 5 mmHg increase in diastolic BP was associated with a 0.17 mmHg increase in IOP in pooled analyses. Yet, the relation between systemic HTN and POAG is not straightforward and suffers from a lack of longitudinal data. Overall, a modest adverse relation between systemic hypertension and POAG was noted in cross-sectional (pooled RR = 1.24; 95% CI: 1.06-1.44; n = 15 studies) but not in case-control studies (pooled RR = 1.08; 95% CI: 0.92-1.28; n = 9 studies) or longitudinal studies (pooled RR = 1.05; 95% CI: 0.69-1.59; n = 2 studies). In terms of dosage of BP, pooled analyses revealed that for every 10 mmHg increase in systolic BP there was a 1% increased risk of POAG (95% CI: 1.00-1.03) but the results for diastolic BP were not statistically significant (pooled RR = 1.02; 95% CI: 0.99-1.04). Results from two studies found no association between systemic HTN and the normal tension variant of POAG where the predominate known IOP measurements are < 22 mmHg (pooled RR = 0.94; 95% CI: 0.56-1.59).

In a prospective study of female and male health professionals that post-dates the meta-analytical literature syntheses, there was a positive association between repeated self-reported measures of BP and incident POAG, whereby every 5 mmHg rise in mean arterial pressure was associated with a 5% increased risk of disease in a multivariable model (OR = 1.05; 95% CI: 1.10-1.09). Yet in the same population, self-reported untreated HTN was not a risk factor for POAG (OR = 1.03; 95% CI: 0.88-1.21).[70]

Overall, while higher BPs are associated with higher IOP, there may be a modest association between systemic HTN and POAG, particularly the high-tension variant. When 16 studies with considerable homogeneity were considered, the pooled RR of the high-tension variant of POAG was 1.22 (95% CI: 1.08-1.37). Among 60 studies with substantial heterogeneity, the pooled RR of POAG overall was 1.16 (95% CI: 1.05-1.28).

B. Treatment of systemic hypertension

It is possible that treatment of systemic HTN could modify the risk of POAG. In considering this matter one must account for the type of BP treatment (diet, drugs, type of drugs) and effectiveness of treatment. In the European Glaucoma Prevention Study, a placebo-controlled trial of dorzolamide 2% bid versus placebo for the treatment of ocular hypertension, diuretic use was a strong inter-current risk factor for the conversion to POAG.[71] In the Blue Mountains Eye Study, HTN that was treated but still regarded as uncontrolled (systolic BP ≥ 160 mmHg or diastolic BP ≥ 95 mmHg despite treatment) was a strong risk factor for OAG, while untreated HTN (BP ≥ 160/95 mmHg) only showed a non-significant trend in the same direction (multivariate adjusted OR = 1.35; 95% CI: 0.75- 2.46).[72] In the Egna-Neumarkt study, where HTN was adversely associated with POAG (OR = 1.7, 95% CI: 1.0-2.9), taking antihypertensive medications was not significantly associated with risk POAG risk (OR=1.3; 95% CI: 0.8-2.3).[73] In the Nurses' Health Study and Health Professionals Follow-up Study, treatment of HTN with diuretics, or with other drugs was not related to incident POAG.[70] Similarly, in the Thessaloniki Eye Study pharmacological treatment of systemic hypertension was not associated with POAG (OR = 1.20; 95% CI: 0.75-1.91).[74] However, when the association of POAG with diastolic OPP was examined in those with and without antihypertensive treatment (stratifying the analysis by perfusion pressure status), the association was confirmed only in subjects who were using antihypertensive treatment (OR = 0.78 per 10 mmHg; 95% CI:0.62-0.97, P = .028). These findings closely relate to those from a previous Thessaloniki Eye Study report.[75] Based on the above, antihypertensive treatment was not an independent risk factor for glaucoma in the Thessaloniki Eye Study; however, low diastolic OPP as a result of antihypertensive treatment was associated with increased risk of POAG. Thus, there is some evidence that treatment for systemic hypertension may be a modifier in the association between BP and glaucoma, and OPP and glaucoma.

Cup-disc ratio is a structural optic nerve parameter that represents an important glaucoma-related trait. In the Thessaloniki Eye Study, a diastolic BP < 90 mmHg that resulted from antihypertensive therapy was associated with increased cupping assessed by Heidelberg Retinal Tomography among non-glaucomatous subjects.[75] Currently, based on available data, how the treatment of HTN impacts the development of POAG remains unclear.

C. Hypotension

BP tends to undergo a physiologic dip at night, but there are limited data comparing these nocturnal dips between POAG patients and controls. For example, one study that included 38 POAG patients, 46 normal-tension glaucoma patients and 11 controls, found more nocturnal dips in BP in glaucoma patients, but this finding was limited to 36 glaucoma patients with progressive visual field loss vs. the stable glaucoma patients.[76] Another clinic-based study from Malaysia found lower night time systolic BP (124.4 ± 19 mmHg vs. 131.8 ± 15.9 mm Hg; p = 0.01) and lower night time diastolic BP (73.3 ± 8.6 mmHg vs 76.2 ± 8.3 mmHg; p=0.05) in 72 NTG patients versus 55 controls using a model adjusting for age and presence of HTN.[77] While low BP is widely touted as a risk factor for POAG, particularly in cases where IOP at presentation is not high, the evidence for this statement is scarce. The Barbados Eye Study failed to find an adverse relation between systolic BP ≤ 110 mmHg or diastolic BP ≤ 71 mmHg (multivariate OR = 1.3; 95% CI: 0.7-2.4) and incident OAG compared to a systolic BP > 153 mmHg or diastolic BP > 90 mmHg.[78] The Singapore Eye Study represents one of the few studies that provide a statistically significant adverse association between low BP and POAG. Compared to the highest quartile of diastolic BP, the lowest quartile of diastolic BP was adversely associated with POAG (OR = 1.71; 95% CI: 1.04-2.96).[69] In the Early Manifest Glaucoma Trial, a randomized clinical trial of topical beta blocker treatment plus laser trabeculoplasty versus observation in relation to OAG disease progression, lower systolic BP ($\leq$ 125 mmHg) was associated with lower risk of progression (Hazards Ratio = 0.46; 95% CI, 0.21-1.02) but this result was not statistically significant.26 It should be mentioned that OAG in this study also included exfoliation glaucoma patients.

In total five studies have evaluated diurnal and nocturnal systolic and diastolic BP variation in POAG patients with progressive versus stable visual field defects. None of these studies were masked and the designation of visual field stability was made retrospectively. A meta-analysis of these studies found no differences in systolic or diastolic BP during the day or during the night in POAG patients with progressive versus stable visual fields.[79] However, the pooled OR of worsening visual field loss among POAG patients with nocturnal dips of systolic or diastolic BP > 10% was 3.32 (95% CI: 1.84-6.00) and 2.09 (95% CI: 1.20-3.04), respectively.

The evidence for increased incidence of nocturnal dips in BP in POAG versus controls is lacking and, overall, the evidence that lower BP contributes to POAG is surprisingly weak.

5.1.2.2. Ocular perfusion pressure

Intuitively it seems logical that a measure of BP minus IOP would be an indicator of the perfusion pressure at the optic nerve head. Various parameters of ocular perfusion pressure are:

- Systolic ocular perfusion pressure (OPP) = systolic BP – IOP
- Diastolic OPP = Diastolic BP - IOP
- Mean OPP = (Diastolic BP + 1/3 (Systolic BP – Diastolic BP)) – IOP

The first population-based study to show a strong inverse relation between OPP and POAG was the Baltimore Eye Study.[80] These findings have been reproduced in other studies,[8,73,74] including a study using incident POAG cases.[78] Moreover, post-hoc analyses of two randomized clinical trials indicated that lower OPP was associated with OAG disease progression.[26,81] Given that the relation between BP and POAG is complex but there is a positive trend toward higher BP and POAG, one must wonder if the relation between lower OPP and POAG is driven mostly by higher IOP. Along these lines, in the Rotterdam Eye Study, the inverse relation between mean OPP and incident POAG became insignificant after adjustment for IOP.[82] Alternatively, since glaucomatous optic neuropathy occurs across the spectrum of both IOP and BP in POAG, the concept of OPP playing an important role in POAG may be of central importance. Finally, the real ocular perfusion is modulated by the functionality of the autoregulatory system and not merely by a simple mathematical distillation of BP and IOP data. In fact, Khawaja and colleagues have argued that when the relation between OPP and POAG is unadjusted for IOP, the effect of IOP predominates, and when such adjustment is performed, the resulting model reflects the relation between BP and POAG.[83] They have suggested that it is time to abandon using parameters like BP-IOP with or without adjustment for IOP as a surrogate for OPP in glaucoma research. Currently, there is insufficient evidence that consideration should be given to ocular perfusion pressure during clinical care of subjects with glaucoma.

5.1.2.3. Vascular dysregulation

All tissue beds require an autoregulatory mechanism that allows for proper delivery of nutrients in the face of varying perfusion pressures and metabolic activity. Vascular dysregulation can be broadly defined as the inability to regulate blood flow at an appropriate level to meet the local physiological needs within a tissue bed. There is considerable evidence from multiple sources that blood flow is dysregulated in POAG. An inability to regulate blood flow in POAG has been demonstrated in various ocular vascular beds, including the choroidal vasculature,[84,85] the optic nerve head circulation,[86,87] retinal vessels,[88-90] and perifoveal capillaries[91] using a variety of experimental paradigms. The autoregulatory abnormalities detected occurred in both the high-tension and normal-tension variant of POAG and extends outside ocular tissue. For example, Quill and colleagues found that digital blood flow responses to either hot or cold stimuli were reduced compared to age-matched controls.[92] These findings are consistent with work by Gasser and Flamer, who found that nailfold capillary blood velocity was more likely to come to a complete standstill after cold provocation in NTG patients.[93]

5.1.2.4. Nailbed capillary

The nailbed contains elongated, inverted U-shaped capillaries that are easily visualized with inexpensive microscopic techniques. Nailfold capillary microscopy may provide alternative insights into systemic vascular dysregulation and hint at the type of microvascular abnormalities that might occur in the optic nerve head capillary bed, which is far more intricate and more challenging to assess. Two cross-sectional studies showed morphological abnormalities (nailbed hemorrhages and large avascular zones) in POAG patients with history of normal and high IOP using multivariable analysis.[94,95] A multisite US study was unable to find a relation between nailfold capillary morphological abnormality and POAG disease severity. No longitudinal studies of nailfold capillary morphological change and glaucoma are available at this time. Therefore, it is unclear whether nailfold capillary abnormality might be a vascular biomarker specific to POAG.

5.1.2.5. Sleep apnea

In obstructive sleep apnea (OSA) repetitive partial or complete upper airway obstruction during sleep produces markedly reduced oxygen saturation levels. Ocular diseases where relations to OSA are suspected include floppy eyelid syndrome, keratoconus, non-arteritic ischemic optic neuropathy and glaucoma. Some studies that have evaluated OAS and glaucoma did not specify the type of glaucoma analyzed. Two small case-control studies found significant adverse associations between OSA and OAG.[96,97] In contrast, a large cohort study derived from a de-identified database did not find any relation between OSA and OAG.[98] A meta-analysis of these studies did not find an association between sleep apnea and OAG (pooled OR = 1.01; 95% CI: 0.97-1.04).[99] Snoring is felt to be a surrogate of OSA and in the Beijing Eye Study this attribute was not associated with OAG.[100] In assessing OSA and OAG one must also account for the effect of continuous positive airway pressure (CPAP), which on one hand may raise IOP101 but on the other may improve blood oxygen levels during sleep. It should be noted that when 'glaucoma' overall[99] or nerve fiber layer thickness[102] is considered as the outcome, a fairly robust adverse relation with OSA is reported in pooled analyses. This suggests that there are glaucoma subtypes for which OSA plays an important role in the generation of glaucomatous damage.

5.1.3. Endocrine System

Jonathan G. Crowston, Sameh Mosaed, Arthur J. Sit

The endocrine system can have a significant effect on intraocular pressure and glaucoma. The effect of glucocorticoids on IOP is very well characterized and will not be discussed in this section. However, multiple other hormones have been suggested as either protective or risk factors for the development of glaucoma.

5.1.3.1. Diabetes and glaucoma[103-112]

Numerous studies investigating the relationship between open-angle glaucoma (OAG) and diabetes mellitus have resulted in conflicting results. However, many of these studies have relied on patient self-reporting of either the glaucoma or the diabetes diagnosis, and did not always distinguish between POAG and NVG. More recent studies with clearer definitions of glaucoma and diabetes seem to indicate that diabetes increases the risk of glaucoma. Also, there may be an effect from diabetes on corneal biomechanical properties, impacting the accuracy of IOP measurements. Taken together, there does seem to be more evidence supporting a correlation between diabetes and POAG, although this is a weaker association than some of the other well-established risk factors such as family history, age, and IOP. In a recent meta-analysis of 47 studies including 2,981,342 individuals from 16 countries, diabetes, diabetes duration, and fasting glucose levels were associated with a significantly increased risk of glaucoma, and diabetes and fasting glucose levels were associated with slightly higher IOP. However, there was substantial heterogeneity in the methods and quality of the original studies. Further studies are needed to determine the magnitude and significance of this association.

5.1.3.2. Thyroid system and glaucoma[14,113-116]

Thyroid orbitopathy is associated with elevation of IOP consequent to mechanical forces exerted by stiff and enlarged extraocular muscles. This can lead to transient IOP elevation with eye movement, in particular up-gaze. Chronic IOP elevation can result from elevated episcleral venous pressure.[113] A number of population studies have revealed a weak but positive association between OAG and thyroid disease. Relative risk ratios generally show a weak association, but the number of glaucoma and thyroid patients in these studies is generally low while thyroid disease diagnosis is often based on self-reported history.[14,114,115] In a retrospective follow-up study of 257 hypothyroidism patients and 2056 controls, hypothyroidism patients were found to have a 1.78-fold (95% confidence interval [CI], 1.04-3.06) greater risk of developing OAG than the comparison cohort, after adjusting for age, gender, monthly income, urbanization level, and comorbid medical disorders. This association remained significant in untreated hypothyroidism patients (adjusted hazard ratio [HR], 2.37; 95% CI, 1.10-5.09) and became statistically nonsignificant in patients treated with levothyroxine (adjusted HR, 1.73; 95% CI, 0.89-3.38). Further studies are needed to determine the association of thyroid disease with glaucoma risk.

5.1.3.3. Sex hormones and glaucoma[117-122]

The effect of sex hormones on IOP and glaucoma has been investigated in numerous epidemiologic studies. Most of this work has focused on the effect in post-menopausal women. Current evidence suggests that the reduction of estrogen in post-menopausal women increases the risk of developing glaucoma. Hormone replacement therapy may reduce IOP and the risk of glaucoma in post-menopausal women. However, bilateral oophorectomy may also increase the risk of glaucoma if performed at an early age, but estrogen replacement does not appear to decrease the risk. In contrast, there is some evidence that the use of oral contraceptives may result in an increased risk of glaucoma. In a cross-sectional study of 3406 female participants from the 2005 to 2008 National Health and Nutrition Examination Survey, those with ≥ three years of oral contraceptive use had greater odds (odds ratio, 1.94; 95% confidence interval, 1.22-3.07) of self-reported glaucoma or ocular hypertension.

5.1.3.4. Other hormones[123,124]

Other hormones including erythropoietin and vasopressin have been found in elevated levels in the aqueous humor of glaucoma patients, and may have acute effects on IOP. However, there is currently a lack of clinical or epidemiologic evidence to support a role for these hormones in glaucoma pathogenesis.

5.1.4. CNS

Based on the anatomy of the optic nerve head with the optic nerve being surrounded by optic nerve meninges and imbedded into the orbital cerebrospinal fluid (CSF), it is apparent that the orbital cerebrospinal fluid pressure (CSFP) is a major determinant of the trans-lamina cribrosa pressure difference.[125,126] It has also been suggested that it is the trans-lamina cribrosa pressure difference, and not the transcorneal pressure difference (which is measured by tonometry), which is the primary pressure parameter in the physiology and pathophysiology of the optic nerve head. In view of the so called normal-pressure-glaucoma, it may be seductive to assume that in these patients the orbital CSFP may be abnormally low, so that in the presence of a normal IOP the trans-lamina cribrosa pressure difference is elevated. Clinical pilot studies and experimental monkey studies have corroborated this hypothesis.[127,128] Some patients with normal-pressure glaucoma, as compared to patients with high-pressure glaucoma and as compared to a control group, showed abnormally low lumbar CSFP measurements.[127] In experimental studies, the lowering of CSFP in monkeys resulted in the development of optic nerve damage.[128] However, it remained unclear whether the observed damage was typical glaucomatous optic neuropathy. The fact that normal-pressure glaucoma is IOP-related could explain why the appearance of the optic nerve head in patients with high-pressure glaucoma and in patients with normal-pressure glaucoma can be strikingly similar. Conversely, the optic nerve head morphology shows marked differences between patients with vascular induced non-glaucomatous optic nerve damage and patients with normal-pressure glaucoma. Considering the orbital CSFP into the physiology of the optic nerve head could also explain that the IOP is allowed to increase in supine position since simultaneously the CSFP elevates.[129] It has remained unclear whether time associated parameters in the trans-lamina relationship between IOP and orbital CSFP may also be of importance.[130] Experimental studies have suggested that the pressure wave coming from the heart first arrives in the CSFP and then in the eye. It could indicate that the trans-lamina cribrosa pressure difference undulates within a pulse cycle. It may theoretically be of importance to allow the retrograde axoplasmic flow to enter the eye. If indeed the trans-lamina cribrosa pressure difference physiologically undulates, any change in timing could lead to a pathological situation, even if the pressures on both sides of the lamina cribrosa are normal. Another aspect is the blood perfusion inside the lamina cribrosa. If the pressure on both sides of the lamina cribrosa is elevated so that the trans-lamina cribrosa pressure difference is normal, the increased pressure tissue in the lamina cribrosa could lead to a compression of the blood capillaries within the lamina cribrosa and to an impediment of blood perfusion.

In summary, there is some evidence that the trans-lamina cribrosa pressure differences (IOP minus orbital cerebrospinal fluid pressure) may contribute to optic nerve pathology. However, there is insufficient evidence to determine whether low orbital cerebrospinal fluid pressure is a risk factor for the development of POAG.

5.1.5. Nutritional Status

Alternative approaches to treatment of glaucoma and their understanding are

5. Mitchell P, Smith W, Attebo K, Healey PR. Prevalence of open-angle glaucoma in Australia. The Blue Mountains Eye Study. Ophthalmology 1996;103(10):1661-1669.
6. Leske MC, Connell AM, Schachat AP, Hyman L. The Barbados Eye Study. Prevalence of open angle glaucoma. Arch Ophthalmol 1994;112(6):821-829.
7. Weih LM, Nanjan M, McCarty CA, Taylor HR. Prevalence and predictors of open-angle glaucoma: results from the visual impairment project. Ophthalmology 2001;108(11):1966-1972.
8. Quigley HA, West SK, Rodriguez J, et al. The prevalence of glaucoma in a population-based study of Hispanic subjects: Proyecto VER. Arch Ophthalmol 2001;119(12):1819-1826.
9. Dandona L, Dandona R, Srinivas M, et al. Open-angle glaucoma in an urban population in southern India: the Andhra Pradesh eye disease study. Ophthalmology 2000;107(9):1702-1709.
10. Iwase A, Suzuki Y, Araie M, et al.; the Tajimi Study Group, Japan Glaucoma Society. The prevalence of primary open-angle glaucoma in Japanese: the Tajimi Study. Ophthalmology 2004;111(9):1641-1648.
11. Varma R, Ying-Lai M, Francis BA, et al.; the Los Angeles Latino Eye Study Group. Prevalence of open-angle glaucoma and ocular hypertension in Latinos: the Los Angeles Latino Eye Study. Ophthalmology 2004;111(8):1439-1448.
12. Topouzis F, Wilson MR, Harris A, et al. Prevalence of open-angle glaucoma in Greece: the Thessaloniki Eye Study. Am J Ophthalmol 2007;144(4):511-519.
13. Shen SY, Wong TY, Foster PJ, et al. The prevalence and types of glaucoma in Malay people: the Singapore Malay Eye Study. Invest Ophthalmol Vis Sci 2008;49(9):3846-3851.
14. Kim M, Kim TW, Park KH, Kim JM. Risk factors for primary open-angle glaucoma in South Korea: the Namil study. Jpn J Ophthalmol 2012;56(4):324-329.
15. Wang YX, Xu L, Yang H, Jonas JB. Prevalence of glaucoma in North China: the Beijing Eye Study. Am J Ophthalmol 2010;150(6):917-924.
16. Casson RJ, Newland HS, Muecke J, et al. Prevalence of glaucoma in rural Myanmar: the Meiktila Eye Study. Br J Ophthalmol 2007;91(6):710-714.
17. Tham YC, Li X, Wong TY, et al. Global prevalence of glaucoma and projections of glaucoma burden through 2040: a systematic review and meta-analysis. Ophthalmology 2014;121(11):2081-2090.
18. de Voogd S, Ikram MK, Wolfs RC, et al. Incidence of open-angle glaucoma in a general elderly population: the Rotterdam Study. Ophthalmology 2005;112(9):1487-1493.
19. Mukesh BN, McCarty CA, Rait JL, Taylor HR. Five-year incidence of open-angle glaucoma: the visual impairment project. Ophthalmology 2002;109(6):1047-1051.
20. Leske MC, Connell AM, Wu SY, et al. Incidence of open-angle glaucoma: the Barbados Eye Studies. The Barbados Eye Studies Group. Arch Ophthalmol 2001;119(1):89-95.
21. Leske MC, Wu SY, Honkanen R, et al.; the Barbados Eye Studies Group. Nine-year incidence of open-angle glaucoma in the Barbados Eye Studies. Ophthalmology 2007;114(6):1058-1064.
22. Broman AT, Quigley HA, West SK, et al. Estimating the rate of progressive visual field damage in those with open-angle glaucoma, from cross-sectional data. Invest Ophthalmol Vis Sci 2008;49(1):66-76.
23. Ocular Hypertension Treatment Study Group; European Glaucoma Prevention Study Group; Gordon MO, Torri V, Miglior S, et al. Validated prediction model for the development of primary open-angle glaucoma in individuals with ocular hypertension. Ophthalmology 2007;114(1):10-19.

24. Nouri-Mahdavi K, Hoffman D, Coleman AL, et al.; Advanced Glaucoma Intervention Study. Predictive factors for glaucomatous visual field progression in the Advanced Glaucoma Intervention Study. Ophthalmology 2004;111(9):1627-1635.
25. Musch DC, Gillespie BW, Lichter PR, Niziol LM, Janz NK; CIGTS Study Investigators. Visual field progression in the Collaborative Initial Glaucoma Treatment Study the impact of treatment and other baseline factors. Ophthalmology 2009;116(2):200-207.
26. Leske MC, Heijl A, Hyman L, et al.; EMGT Group. Predictors of long-term progression in the early manifest glaucoma trial. Ophthalmology 2007;114(11):1965-1972.
27. Rudnicka AR, Mt-Isa S, Owen CG, Cook DG, Ashby D. Variations in primary open-angle glaucoma prevalence by age, gender, and race: a Bayesian meta-analysis. Invest Ophthalmol Vis Sci 2006;47(10):4254-4261.
28. Heijl A, Leske MC, Bengtsson B, et al.; the Early Manifest Glaucoma Trial Group. Reduction of intraocular pressure and glaucoma progression: results from the Early Manifest Glaucoma Trial. Arch Ophthalmol 2002;120(10):1268-1279.
29. Kass MA, Gordon MO, Gao F, et al.; the Ocular Hypertension Treatment Study Group. Delaying treatment of ocular hypertension: the ocular hypertension treatment study. Arch Ophthalmol 2010;128(3):276-287.
30. Hoevenaars JG, Schouten JS, van den Borne B, Beckers HJ, Webers CA. Socioeconomic differences in glaucoma patients' knowledge, need for information and expectations of treatments. Acta Ophthalmol Scand 2006;84(1):84-91.
31. Attebo K, Mitchell P, Cumming R, Smith W. Knowledge and beliefs about common eye diseases. Aust N Z J Ophthalmol 1997;25(4):283-287.
32. Zhang X, Beckles GL, Chou CF, et al. Socioeconomic disparity in use of eye care services among US adults with age-related eye diseases: National Health Interview Survey, 2002 and 2008. JAMA Ophthalmol 2013;131(9):1198-1206.
33. Ko YC, Hwang DK, Chen WT, Lee CC, Liu CJ. Impact of Socioeconomic Status on the Diagnosis of Primary Open-Angle Glaucoma and Primary Angle Closure Glaucoma: A Nationwide Population-Based Study in Taiwan. PLoS One 2016;11(2):e0149698.
34. Hennis A, Wu SY, Nemesure B, Honkanen R, Leske MC; the Barbados Eye Studies Group. Awareness of incident open-angle glaucoma in a population study: the Barbados Eye Studies. Ophthalmology 2007;114(10):1816-1821.
35. Topouzis F, Coleman AL, Harris A, et al. Factors associated with undiagnosed open-angle glaucoma: the Thessaloniki Eye Study. Am J Ophthalmol 2008;145(2):327-335.
36. Ratnarajan G, Coombes E, Jones A, Parker M, Bourne R. The equity profile of an enhanced optometry scheme. Ophthalmic Physiol Opt 2015;35(2):243-244.
37. Buys YM, Jin YP; the Canadian Glaucoma Risk Factor Study Group. Socioeconomic status as a risk factor for late presentation of glaucoma in Canada. Can J Ophthalmol 2013;48(2):83-87.
38. Ng WS, Agarwal PK, Sidiki S, et al. The effect of socio-economic deprivation on severity of glaucoma at presentation. Br J Ophthalmol 2010;94(1):85-87.
39. Fraser S, Bunce C, Wormald R, Brunner E. Deprivation and late presentation of glaucoma: case-control study. BMJ 2001;322(7287):639-643.
40. Thorleifsson G, Walters GB, Hewitt AW, et al. Common variants near CAV1 and CAV2 are associated with primary open-angle glaucoma. Nat Genet 2010;42(10):906-909.
41. Burdon KP, Macgregor S, Hewitt AW, et al. Genome-wide association study identifies susceptibility loci for open angle glaucoma at TMCO1 and CDKN2B-AS1. Nat Genet 2011;43(6):574-578.

42. Wiggs JL, Yaspan BL, Hauser MA, et al. Common variants at 9p21 and 8q22 are associated with increased susceptibility to optic nerve degeneration in glaucoma. PLoS Genet 2012;8(4):e1002654.
43. Gharahkhani P, Burdon KP, Fogarty R, et al. Common variants near ABCA1, AFAP1 and GMDS confer risk of primary open-angle glaucoma. Nat Genet 2014;46(10):1120-1125.
44. Hysi PG, Cheng CY, Springelkamp H, et al. Genome-wide analysis of multi-ancestry cohorts identifies new loci influencing intraocular pressure and susceptibility to glaucoma. Nat Genet 2014;46(10):1126-1130.
45. Chen Y, Lin Y, Vithana EN, et al. Common variants near ABCA1 and in PMM2 are associated with primary open-angle glaucoma. Nat Genet 2014;46(10):1115-1119.
46. Trikha S, Saffari E, Nongpiur M, et al. A Genetic Variant in TGFBR3-CDC7 Is Associated with Visual Field Progression in Primary Open-Angle Glaucoma Patients from Singapore. Ophthalmology 2015;122(12):2416-2422.
47. Bailey JN, Loomis SJ, Kang JH, et al. Genome-wide association analysis identifies TXNRD2, ATXN2 and FOXC1 as susceptibility loci for primary open-angle glaucoma. Nat Genet 2016;48(2):189-194.
48. Stone EM, Fingert JH, Alward WL, et al. Identification of a gene that causes primary open angle glaucoma. Science 1997;275(5300):668-670.
49. Stoilova D, Child A, Trifan OC, et al. Localization of a locus (GLC1B) for adult-onset primary open angle glaucoma to the 2cen-q13 region. Genomics 1996;36(1):142-150.
50. Wirtz MK, Samples JR, Kramer PL, et al. Mapping a gene for adult-onset primary open-angle glaucoma to chromosome 3q. Am J Hum Genet 1997;60(2):296-304.
51. Trifan OC, Traboulsi EI, Stoilova D, et al. A third locus (GLC1D) for adult-onset primary open-angle glaucoma maps to the 8q23 region. Am J Ophthalmol 1998;126(1):17-28.
52. Rezaie T, Child A, Hitchings R, et al. Adult-onset primary open-angle glaucoma caused by mutations in optineurin. Science 2002;295(5557):1077-1079.
53. Pasutto F, Keller KE, Weisschuh N, et al. Variants in ASB10 are associated with open-angle glaucoma. Hum Mol Genet 2012;21(6):1336-1349.
54. Monemi S, Spaeth G, DaSilva A, et al. Identification of a novel adult-onset primary open-angle glaucoma (POAG) gene on 5q22.1. Hum Mol Genet 2005;14(6):725-733.
55. Suriyapperuma SP, Child A, Desai T, et al. A new locus (GLC1H) for adult-onset primary open-angle glaucoma maps to the 2p15-p16 region. Arch Ophthalmol 2007;125(1):86-92.
56. Woodroffe A, Krafchak CM, Fuse N, et al. Ordered subset analysis supports a glaucoma locus at GLC1I on chromosome 15 in families with earlier adult age at diagnosis. Exp Eye Res 2006;82(6):1068-1074.
57. Wiggs JL, Lynch S, Ynagi G, et al. A genomewide scan identifies novel early-onset primary open-angle glaucoma loci on 9q22 and 20p12. Am J Hum Genet 2004;74(6):1314-1320.
58. Sherwin JC, Hewitt AW, Bennett SL, et al. Primary open angle glaucoma in subjects harbouring the predicted GLC1L haplotype reveals a normotensive phenotype. Clin Experiment Ophthalmol 2009;37(2):201-207.
59. Fan BJ, Ko WC, Wang DY, et al. Fine mapping of new glaucoma locus GLC1M and exclusion of neuregulin 2 as the causative gene. Mol Vis 2007;13:779-784.
60. Aragon-Martin JA, Ritch R, Liebmann J, et al. Evaluation of LOXL1 gene polymorphisms in exfoliation syndrome and exfoliation glaucoma. Mol Vis 2008;14:533-541.
61. Pasutto F, Matsumoto T, Mardin CY, et al. Heterozygous NTF4 mutations impairing neurotrophin-4 signaling in patients with primary open-angle glaucoma. Am J Hum Genet 2009;85(4):447-456.

62. Fingert JH, Robin AL, Stone JL, et al. Copy number variations on chromosome 12q14 in patients with normal tension glaucoma. Hum Mol Genet 2011;20(12):2482-2494.
63. Porter LF, Urquhart JE, O'Donoghue E, et al. Identification of a novel locus for autosomal dominant primary open angle glaucoma on 4q35.1-q35.2. Invest Ophthalmol Vis Sci 2011;52(11):7859-7865.
64. Stoilov I, Akarsu AN, Sarfarazi M. Identification of three different truncating mutations in cytochrome P4501B1 (CYP1B1) as the principal cause of primary congenital glaucoma (Buphthalmos) in families linked to the GLC3A locus on chromosome 2p21. Hum Mol Genet 1997;6(4):641-647.
65. Akarsu AN, Turacli ME, Aktan SG, et al. A second locus (GLC3B) for primary congenital glaucoma (Buphthalmos) maps to the 1p36 region. Hum Mol Genet 1996;5(8):1199-1203.
66. Narooie-Nejad M, Paylakhi SH, Shojaee S, et al. Loss of function mutations in the gene encoding latent transforming growth factor beta binding protein 2, LTBP2, cause primary congenital glaucoma. Hum Mol Genet 2009;18(20):3969-3977.
67. Zhao D, Cho J, Kim MH, Guallar E. The association of blood pressure and primary open-angle glaucoma: a meta-analysis. Am J Ophthalmol 2014;158(3):615-627.
68. Bae HW, Lee N, Lee HS, et al. Systemic hypertension as a risk factor for open-angle glaucoma: a meta-analysis of population-based studies. PLoS One 2014;9(9):e108226.
69. Zheng Y, Wong TY, Mitchell P, et al. Distribution of ocular perfusion pressure and its relationship with open-angle glaucoma: the Singapore Malay Eye Study. Invest Ophthalmol Vis Sci 2010;51(7):3399-3404.
70. Kang JH, Loomis SJ, Rosner BA, Wiggs JL, Pasquale LR. Comparison of Risk Factor Profiles for Primary Open-Angle Glaucoma Subtypes Defined by Pattern of Visual Field Loss: A Prospective Study. Invest Ophthalmol Vis Sci 2015;56(4):2439-2448.
71. Miglior S, Torri V, Zeyen T, et al.; the EGPS Group. Intercurrent factors associated with the development of open-angle glaucoma in the European glaucoma prevention study. Am J Ophthalmol 2007;144(2):266-275.
72. Mitchell P, Lee AJ, Rochtchina E, Wang JJ. Open-angle glaucoma and systemic hypertension: the blue mountains eye study. J Glaucoma 2004;13(4):319-326.
73. Bonomi L, Marchini G, Marraffa M, et al. Vascular risk factors for primary open angle glaucoma: the Egna-Neumarkt Study. Ophthalmology 2000;107(7):1287-1293.
74. Topouzis F, Wilson MR, Harris A, et al. Association of open-angle glaucoma with perfusion pressure status in the Thessaloniki Eye Study. Am J Ophthalmol 2013;155(5):843-851.
75. Topouzis F, Coleman AL, Harris A, et al. Association of blood pressure status with the optic disk structure in non-glaucoma subjects: the Thessaloniki Eye Study. Am J Ophthalmol 2006;142(1):60-67.
76. Graham SL, Drance SM, Wijsman K, Douglas GR, Mikelberg FS. Ambulatory blood pressure monitoring in glaucoma. The nocturnal dip. Ophthalmology 1995;102(1):61-69.
77. Ramli N, Nurull BS, Hairi NN, Mimiwati Z. Low nocturnal ocular perfusion pressure as a risk factor for normal tension glaucoma. Prev Med 2013;57 Suppl:S47-49.
78. Leske MC, Wu SY, Hennis A, Honkanen R, Nemesure B; the BESs Study Group. Risk factors for incident open-angle glaucoma: the Barbados Eye Studies. Ophthalmology 2008;115(1):85-93.
79. Bowe A, Grünig M, Schubert J, et al. Circadian Variation in Arterial Blood Pressure and Glaucomatous Optic Neuropathy – A Systematic Review and Meta-Analysis. Am J Hypertens 2015;28(9):1077-1082.

80. Tielsch JM, Katz J, Sommer A, Quigley HA, Javitt JC. Hypertension, perfusion pressure, and primary open-angle glaucoma. A population-based assessment. Arch Ophthalmol 1995;113(2):216-221.
81. De Moraes CG, Liebmann JM, Greenfield DS, et al.; the Low-pressure Glaucoma Treatment Study Group. Risk factors for visual field progression in the low-pressure glaucoma treatment study. Am J Ophthalmol 2012;154(4):702-711.
82. Ramdas WD, Wolfs RC, Hofman A, et al. Ocular perfusion pressure and the incidence of glaucoma: real effect or artifact? The Rotterdam Study. Invest Ophthalmol Vis Sci 2011;52(9):6875-6881.
83. Khawaja AP, Crabb DP, Jansonius NM. The role of ocular perfusion pressure in glaucoma cannot be studied with multivariable regression analysis applied to surrogates. Invest Ophthalmol Vis Sci 2013;54(7):4619-4620.
84. Ulrich A, Ulrich C, Barth T, Ulrich WD. Detection of disturbed autoregulation of the peripapillary choroid in primary open angle glaucoma. Ophthalmic Surg Lasers 1996;27(9):746-757.
85. Gugleta K, Orgül S, Hasler PW, et al. Choroidal vascular reaction to hand-grip stress in subjects with vasospasm and its relevance in glaucoma. Invest Ophthalmol Vis Sci 2003;44(4):1573-1580.
86. Fuchsjäger-Mayrl G, Wally B, Georgopoulos M, et al. Ocular blood flow and systemic blood pressure in patients with primary open-angle glaucoma and ocular hypertension. Invest Ophthalmol Vis Sci 2004;45(3):834-839.
87. Okuno T, Sugiyama T, Kojima S, Nakajima M, Ikeda T. Diurnal variation in microcirculation of ocular fundus and visual field change in normal-tension glaucoma. Eye (Lond) 2004;18(7):697-702.
88. Evans DW, Harris A, Garrett M, Chung HS, Kagemann L. Glaucoma patients demonstrate faulty autoregulation of ocular blood flow during posture change. Br J Ophthalmol 1999;83(7):809-813.
89. Galambos P, Vafiadis J, Vilchez SE, et al. Compromised autoregulatory control of ocular hemodynamics in glaucoma patients after postural change. Ophthalmology 2006;113(10):1832-1836.
90. Feke GT, Pasquale LR. Retinal blood flow response to posture change in glaucoma patients compared with healthy subjects. Ophthalmology 2008;115(2):246-252.
91. Grunwald JE, Riva CE, Stone RA, Keates EU, Petrig BL. Retinal autoregulation in open-angle glaucoma. Ophthalmology 1984;91(12):1690-1694.
92. Quill B, Henry E, Simon E, O'Brien CJ. Evaluation of the Effect of Hypercapnia on Vascular Function in Normal Tension Glaucoma. Biomed Res Int 2015;2015:418159.
93. Gasser P, Flammer J. Blood-cell velocity in the nailfold capillaries of patients with normal-tension and high-tension glaucoma. Am J Ophthalmol 1991;111(5):585-588.
94. Park HY, Park SH, Oh YS, Park CK. Nail bed hemorrhage: a clinical marker of optic disc hemorrhage in patients with glaucoma. Arch Ophthalmol 2011;129(10):1299-1304.
95. Pasquale LR, Hanyuda A, Ren A, et al. Nailfold Capillary Abnormalities in Primary Open-Angle Glaucoma: A Multisite Study. Invest Ophthalmol Vis Sci 2015;56(12):7021-7028.
96. Bilgin G. Normal-tension glaucoma and obstructive sleep apnea syndrome: a prospective study. BMC Ophthalmol 2014;14:27. doi: 10.1186/1471-2415-14-27.
97. Dong X, Zhang C, Huang P, Du C. Relationship between normal-tension glaucoma and sleep-breathing events. Zhonghua Shiyan Yanke Zazhi/Chinese Journal of Experimental Ophthalmology 2014;32(2):172-177.

98. Stein JD, Kim DS, Mundy KM, et al. The association between glaucomatous and other causes of optic neuropathy and sleep apnea. Am J Ophthalmol 2011;152(6):989-998.
99. Liu S, Lin Y, Liu X. Meta-Analysis of Association of Obstructive Sleep Apnea With Glaucoma. J Glaucoma 2016;25(1):1-7.
100. Wang YX, Xu L, Li JJ, et al. Snoring and glaucoma. PLoS One 2014;9(2):e88949.
101. Kiekens S, Veva De Groot, Coeckelbergh T, et al. Continuous positive airway pressure therapy is associated with an increase in intraocular pressure in obstructive sleep apnea. Invest Ophthalmol Vis Sci 2008;49(3):934-940.
102. Zhao XJ, Yang CC, Zhang JC, et al. Obstructive Sleep Apnea and Retinal Nerve Fiber Layer Thickness: A Meta-analysis. J Glaucoma 2016;25(4):e413-8.
103. Zhou M, Wang W, Huang W, Zhang X. Diabetes mellitus as a risk factor for open-angle glaucoma: a systematic review and meta-analysis. PLoS One 2014;9(8):e102972.
104. Charlson ES, Sankar PS, Miller-Ellis E, et al. The primary open-angle African-American glaucoma genetics study: baseline demographics. Ophthalmology 2015;122(4):711-720.
105. Zhao D, Cho J, Kim MH, Friedman DS, Guallar E. Diabetes, fasting glucose, and the risk of glaucoma: a meta-analysis. Ophthalmology 2015;122(1):72-78.
106. Dielemans I, de Jong PT, Stolk R, et al. Primary open-angle glaucoma, intraocular pressure, and diabetes mellitus in the general elderly population. The Rotterdam Study. Ophthalmology 1996;103(8):1271-1275.
107. Coudrillier B, Pijanka J, Jefferys J, et al. Effects of age and diabetes on scleral stiffness. J Biomech Eng 2015;137(7). doi: 10.1115/1.4029986.
108. Mitchell P, Smith W, Chey T, Healey PR. Open-angle glaucoma and diabetes: the Blue Mountains eye study, Australia. Ophthalmology 1997;104(4):712-718.
109. Bonovas S, Peponis V, Filioussi K. Diabetes mellitus as a risk factor for primary open-angle glaucoma: a meta-analysis. Diabet Med 2004;21(6):609-614.
110. Tielsch JM, Katz J, Quigley HA, et al. Diabetes, intraocular pressure, and primary open-angle glaucoma in the Baltimore Eye Survey. Ophthalmology 1995;102:48-53.
111. Bengtsson B, Heijl A. A long-term prospective study of risk factors for glaucomatous visual field loss in patients with ocular hypertension. J Glaucoma 2005;14:135-138.
112. Chopra V, Varma R, Francis BA, et al. Type 2 diabetes mellitus and the risk of open-angle glaucoma the Los Angeles Latino Eye Study. Los Angeles Latino Eye Study Group. Ophthalmology 2008;115(2):227-232.
113. Haefliger IO, von Arx G, Pimentel AR. Pathophysiology of intraocular pressure increase and glaucoma prevalence in thyroid eye disease: a mini-review. Klin Monatsbl Augenheilkd 2010;227(4):292-293. doi: 10.1055/s-0029-1245199. Epub 2010 Apr 20.
114. Lee AJ, Rochtchina E, Wang JJ, Healey PR, Mitchell P. Open-angle glaucoma and systemic thyroid disease in an older population: The Blue Mountains Eye Study. Eye (Lond) 2004;18(6):600-608.
115. Cross JM, Girkin CA, Owsley C, McGwin G Jr. The association between thyroid problems and glaucoma. Br J Ophthalmol 2008;92(11):1503-1505. doi: 10.1136/bjo.2008.147165.
116. Lin HC, Kang JH, Jiang YD, Ho JD. Hypothyroidism and the risk of developing open-angle glaucoma: a five-year population-based follow-up study. Ophthalmology 2010;117(10):1960-1966.
117. Vajaranant TS, Grossardt BR, Maki PM, et al. Risk of glaucoma after early bilateral oophorectomy. Menopause 2014;21(4):391-398.
118. Pasquale LR, Rosner BA, Hankinson SE, Kang JH. Attributes of female reproductive aging and their relation to primary open-angle glaucoma: a prospective study. J Glaucoma 2007;16(7):598-605.

119. Pasquale LR, Kang JH. Female reproductive factors and primary open-angle glaucoma in the Nurses' Health Study. Eye (Lond) 2011;25(5):633-641.
120. Tint NL, Alexander P, Tint KM, et al. Hormone therapy and intraocular pressure in nonglaucomatous eyes. Menopause 2010;17(1):157-160.
121. Toker E, Yenice O, Temel A. Influence of serum levels of sex hormones on intraocular pressure in menopausal women. J Glaucoma 2003;12(5):436-440.
122. Wang YE, Kakigi C, Barbosa D, et al. Oral Contraceptive Use and Prevalence of Self-Reported Glaucoma or Ocular Hypertension in the United States. Ophthalmology 2016;123(4):729-736.
123. Bogner B, Runge C, Strohmaier C, et al. The effect of vasopressin on ciliary blood flow and aqueous flow. Invest Ophthalmol Vis Sci 2014;21;55(1):396-403.
124. Nassiri N, Nassiri N, Majdi M, et al. Erythropoietin levels in aqueous humor of patients with glaucoma. Mol Vis 2012;18:1991-1995.
125. Morgan WH, Yu DY, Balaratnasingam C. The role of cerebrospinal fluid pressure in glaucoma pathophysiology: the dark side of the optic disc. J Glaucoma 2008;17(5):408-413.
126. Jonas JB, Wang N, Yang D, Ritch R, Panda-Jonas S. Facts and myths of cerebrospinal fluid pressure for the physiology of the eye. Prog Retin Eye Res 2015;46:67-83.
127. Ren R, Jonas JB, Tian G, et al. Cerebrospinal fluid pressure in glaucoma. A prospective study. Ophthalmology 2010;117(2):259-266.
128. Yang D, Fu J, Hou R, et al. Optic neuropathy induced by experimentally reduced cerebrospinal fluid pressure in monkeys. Invest Ophthalmol Vis Sci 2014;55(5):3067-3073.
129. Jasien JV, de Moraes CG, Jonas JB, Ritch R. Rise of intraocular pressure in subjects with and without glaucoma during four common yoga positions. PLoS One 2015;10(12):e0144505.
130. Morgan WH, Lind CR, Kain S, et al. Retinal vein pulsation is in phase with intracranial pressure and not intraocular pressure. Invest Ophthalmol Vis Sci 2012;53(8):4676-4681.
131. Kang JH, Willett WC, Rosner BA, et al. Association of Dietary Nitrate Intake With Primary Open-Angle Glaucoma: A Prospective Analysis From the Nurses' Health Study and Health Professionals Follow-up Study. JAMA Ophthalmol 2016;134(3):294-303.
132. Park SC, De Moraes CG, Teng CC, et al. Initial parafoveal versus peripheral scotomas in glaucoma: risk factors and visual field characteristics. Ophthalmology 2011;118(9):1782-1789.
133. Kang JW, Park B, Cho BJ. Comparison of risk factors for initial central scotoma versus initial peripheral scotoma in normal-tension glaucoma. Korean J Ophthalmol 2015;29(2):102-108.
134. Giaconi JA, Yu F, Stone KL, et al.; Study of Osteoporotic Fractures Research Group. The association of consumption of fruits/vegetables with decreased risk of glaucoma among older African-American women in the study of osteoporotic fractures. Am J Ophthalmol 2012;154(4):635-644.
135. Nguyen CT, Vingrys AJ, Bui BV. Dietary ω-3 deficiency and IOP insult are additive risk factors for ganglion cell dysfunction. J Glaucoma 2013;22(4):269-277.
136. Ramdas WD, Wolfs RC, Kiefte-de Jong JC, et al. Nutrient intake and risk of open-angle glaucoma: the Rotterdam Study. Eur J Epidemiol 2012;27(5):385-393.
137. Kang JH, Pasquale LR, Willett WC, et al. Dietary fat consumption and primary open-angle glaucoma. Am J Clin Nutr 2004;79(5):755-764.
138. Pérez de Arcelus M, Toledo E, Martínez-González MÁ, et al. Omega 3:6 ratio intake and incidence of glaucoma: the SUN cohort. Clin Nutr 2014;33(6):1041-1045.
139. Renard JP, Rouland JF, Bron A, et al. Nutritional, lifestyle and environmental factors in ocular hypertension and primary open-angle glaucoma: an exploratory case-control study. Acta Ophthalmol 2013;91(6):505-513.

140. Yoo TK, Oh E, Hong S. Is vitamin D status associated with open-angle glaucoma? A cross-sectional study from South Korea. Public Health Nutr 2014;17(4):833-843.
141. Wang SY, Singh K, Lin SC. Glaucoma prevalence and the intake of iron and calcium in a population-based study. Curr Eye Res 2013;38(10):1049-1056.
142. Bruhn RL, Stamer WD, Herrygers LA, Levine JM, Noecker RJ. Relationship between glaucoma and selenium levels in plasma and aqueous humour. Br J Ophthalmol 2009;93(9):1155-1158.
143. Pasquale LR, Wiggs JL, Willett WC, Kang JH. The Relationship between caffeine and coffee consumption and exfoliation glaucoma or glaucoma suspect: a prospective study in two cohorts. Invest Ophthalmol Vis Sci 2012;53(10):6427-6433.
144. Kang JH, Loomis SJ, Wiggs JL, Willett WC, Pasquale LR. A prospective study of folate, vitamin B_6, and vitamin B_{12} intake in relation to exfoliation glaucoma or suspected exfoliation glaucoma. JAMA Ophthalmol 2014;132(5):549-559.
145. Paolisso G, Tagliamonte MR, Rizzo MR, et al. Oxidative stress and advancing age: results in healthy centenarians. J Am Geriatr Soc 1998;46(7):833-838.
146. Tezel G. Oxidative stress in glaucomatous neurodegeneration: mechanisms and consequences. Prog Retin Eye Res 2006;25(5):490-513.
147. Lee S, Van Bergen NJ, Kong GY, et al. Mitochondrial dysfunction in glaucoma and emerging bioenergetic therapies. Exp Eye Res 2011;93(2):204-212.
148. Yang XJ, Ge J, Zhuo YH. Role of mitochondria in the pathogenesis and treatment of glaucoma. Chin Med J (Engl) 2013;126(22):4358-4365.
149. Osborne NN, Núñez-Álvarez C, Joglar B, Del Olmo-Aguado S. Glaucoma: Focus on mitochondria in relation to pathogenesis and neuroprotection. Eur J Pharmacol 2016 Apr 14. pii: S0014-2999(16)30243-6.

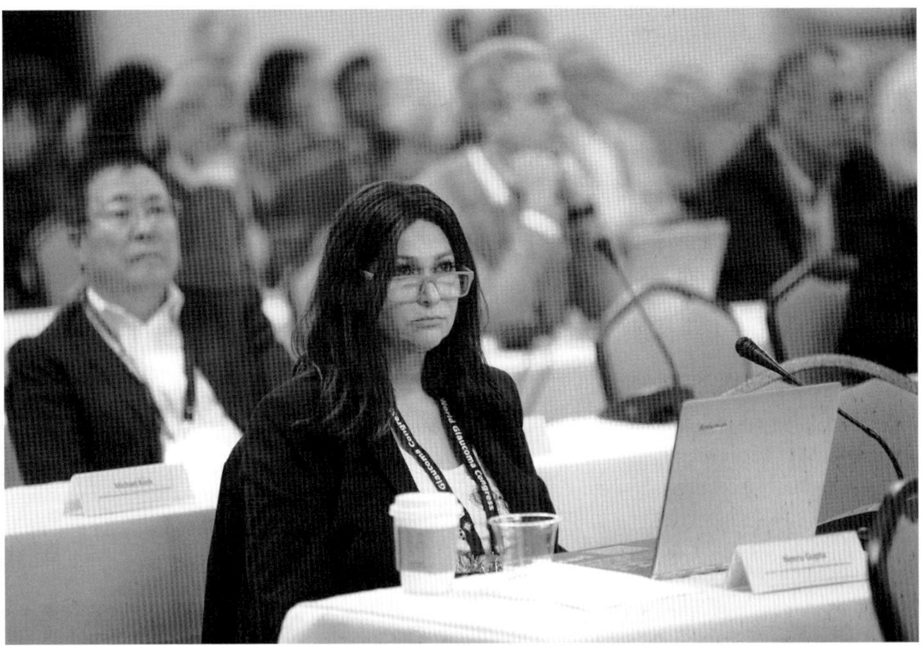

Ningli Wang and Neeru Gupta

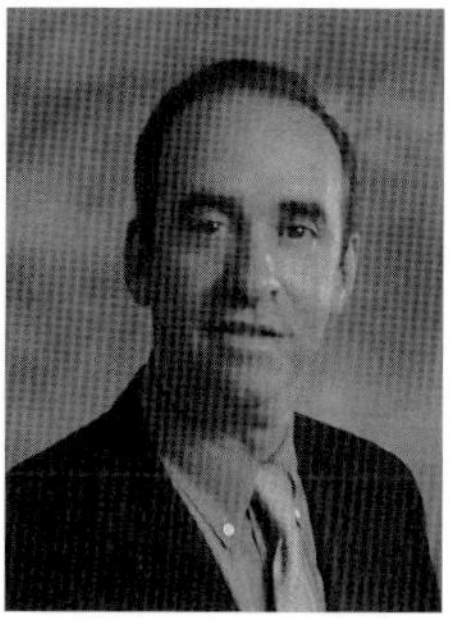
Jeffrey Liebmann

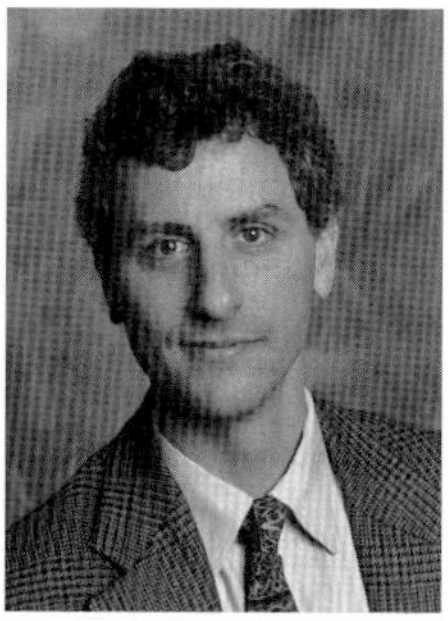
David Friedman

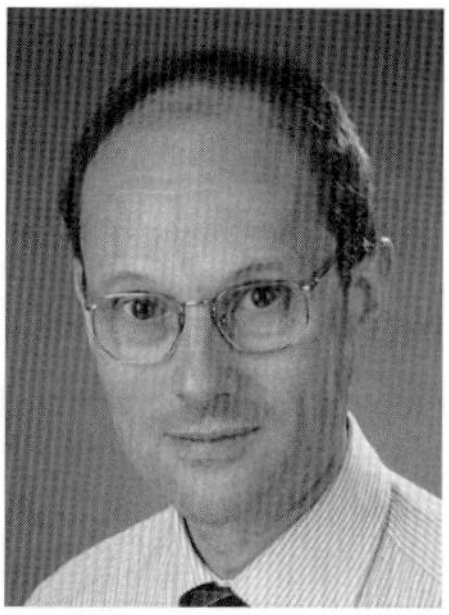
Jost Jonas

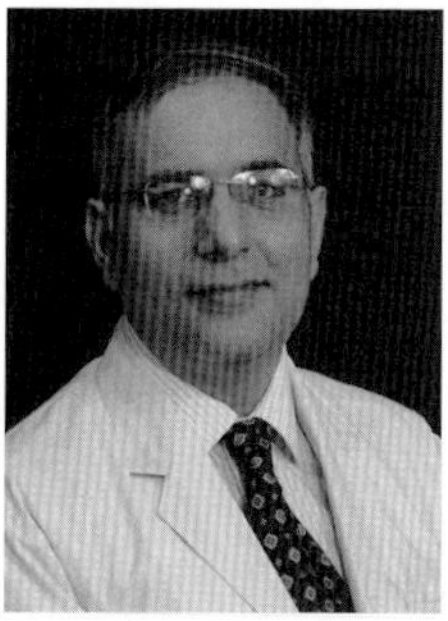
Tanuj Dada

6. SCREENING

Section leader: Jeffrey Liebmann
Section co-leaders: David Friedman, Jost Jonas, Tanuj Dada
Contributors: Eytan Blumenthal, Rupert Bourne, Alain Bron, Anne Louise Coleman, Vital Costa, Paulus de Jong, Murray Fingeret, Ronnie George, Parul Ichhpujani, Dan Kiage, Aravind Krishnadas, Shan Lin, Steven Mansberger, Vinay Nangia, Shamira Perera, Norbert Pfeiffer, Sola Olawoye, G. Chandra Sekhar, Fotis Topouzis

Consensus statements

1. Glaucoma is the leading cause of irreversible blindness worldwide.
   Comment: In some countries, as many as 90% of glaucoma patients remain undiagnosed.
2. Screening everyone for glaucoma is an ideal proposition, but it is not logistically feasible. It would also result in an unacceptably high number of individuals with a false-positive diagnosis of glaucoma.
   Comment: To be effective, screening programs should select participants at substantial risk for glaucoma.
3. The cost-effectiveness of screening for POAG alone has not been demonstrated.
   Comment: Cost-effectiveness for glaucoma may be enhanced when done with other ocular conditions that cause visual impairment, including uncorrected refractive error, cataract, diabetic retinopathy, and age-related macular degeneration.
4. First-degree relatives of individuals with POAG and those with significant risk factors should be examined.

6.1. The magnitude of the problem

Glaucoma is an acquired and progressive optic neuropathy with characteristic optic nerve damage and eventual visual field changes. Individuals with glaucoma

Diagnosis of Primary Open Angle Glaucoma, pp 189-210
Edited by Robert N. Weinreb, David Garway-Heath, Christopher Leung, Felipe Medeiros, Jeffrey Liebmann

Optical Coherence Tomography (OCT): OCT measures reflectance from the retina using a 840 nm light source. The resolution of OCT imaging has dramatically improved from the time domain (TD) machines to the spectral domain (SD) instruments. The current spectral-domain (SD) OCT technology collects up to 55,000 A-scans per second with an axial resolution of 5 μm – a 100-fold improvement over the earlier-generation TD-OCT. Optic nerve head and nerve fiber layer imaging devices allow for simplified screening since the devices frequently can image through an undilated pupil and have automated software to grade the images. However, there are significant cost issues as well as challenges in transporting these devices for outreach screening programs (although portable versions are being developed). Changes in hardware and software over time necessitate repeat validations of the screening effectiveness of the devices.[76] All the devices are affected by cataract to some extent and this has the potential to limit their utility in populations with significant numbers of visually significant cataract.

Li and coworkers have shown that screening for glaucoma in a community-based high-risk population with TD-OCT resulted in moderate sensitivity and high specificity for definitive glaucoma suggesting that the device does not have adequate sensitivity to be used alone but may have utility in excluding subjects from further evaluation.77 OCT currently lacks the necessary diagnostic performance for general population glaucoma screening.

However, SD-OCT has been reported to have higher sensitivity than TD-OCT in glaucoma screening and may have potential for early detection in a high-risk population.[78]

6.8.2.4. Perimetry

Testing of the peripheral visual field can detect vision loss from glaucomatous optic neuropathy. Testing of the visual field can be performed with easily portable devices and efforts are being made to develop tablet-based tests.[73]

Standard Achromatic Perimetry (SAP): Assessing visual fields using the 'reference standard' SAP can be difficult as the reliability of a single measurement may be low; several consistent measurements are needed to establish the presence of defects.

Full-threshold programs are not useful for screening because of the time needed for testing. Scoring Algorithms, such as the Swedish interactive threshold algorithm (SITA) with the Humphrey Field Analyzer(HFA), are faster, but portability of the machine remains an issue. Suprathreshold screening at a limited number of points may be faster yet, but none of the major visual field instruments have distinguished themselves as particularly useful for screening using this method.

Frequency Doubling Perimetry (FDP): FDP uses a stimulus with a high temporal and low spatial frequency to detect visual field defects. It is a portable and easy-to-administer test that does not require specialized testing conditions. The test in screening mode generally takes less than two minutes per eye. The C-20-1 screening test exhibits low sensitivity for the detection of mild loss but high sensitivity for advanced field loss relative to Program 24-2 and the SITA Fast algorithm of the HFA. Sensitivity can be increased by use of the C-20-5 screening protocol. The C-20-5 screening test presents targets at a contrast level that 95% of healthy age-matched subjects would be expected to detect. Screening studies have reported sensitivity and specificity to range from about 80 to 100%, depending on the criteria used and subjects screened.[79]

More recently, Francis *et al.* assessed various parameters in the Los Angeles Latino Eye Study (LALES) both individually and in combination with three historical high-risk parameters – age greater than 65 years, a family history of glaucoma and diabetes.[81] The AUROC for vertical cup to disc ratio was 0.895 for the high-risk group and 0.9 for the entire population, for IOP corresponding AUROC was 0.668 and 0.705. The AUROC for MD and PSD on visual field testing were 0.835 each for any high-risk group. The corresponding AUROC for the entire population was 0.865. The addition of a historical risk factor did not appear to improve diagnostic ability of any of the tests evaluated.

A Cochrane review in 2015 assessed the diagnostic accuracy of HRT, OCT and GDx for diagnosing glaucoma by detecting ONH and RNFL damage and reported that the Nerve Fiber Indicator (NFI) among the GDx parameters yielded the highest accuracy for this device (estimate, 95% confidence interval (CI)) (sensitivity: 0.67, 0.55 to 0.77; specificity: 0.94, 0.92 to 0.95). For HRT measures, the vertical CDR (sensitivity: 0.72, 0.60 to 0.68; specificity: 0.94, 0.92 to 0.95) was similar to other parameters. With OCT, the average RNFL retinal thickness and inferior RNFL thickness were similar (0.72, 0.65 to 0.77; specificity: 0.93, 0.92 to 0.95).[82] The review specifically did not include population-based studies – this is likely to bias the diagnostic ability since the participant profile in clinic-based studies may differ from those in the general population. There are few studies that report the use of the spectral domain OCT as a screening tool in a population.

6.8.2.5. Genetic testing

A number of genetic loci associated with POAG have been identified. Some such as the *GLN368 Stop mutation* in the *Myocilin gene* 'cause disease' while others, such as *Chromosome 7q31 risk allele (rs4236601A)*, contribute to the overall risk for developing disease.[83] However, while the presence of the MYOC mutation is associated with a 90% probability of developing glaucoma these 'disease causing' mutations account for a small proportion (less than 5%) of those with POAG. This low prevalence of 3-5% of the mutation in most populations reduces its utility as a screening test. Differences in the mutation profile between Caucasians and African American POAG patients again make it unlikely that a common set of

Table 1. Summary of Sensitivity, Specificity and DOR and mean interpretable range for Tests Included in the HSROC Meta-analysis Models (adapted from Ervin[73] and Mowatt *et al.*[80])

Test	**Number of Studies**	**Common Cutoff**	**Sensitivity % (95% CrI)**	**Specificity % (95% CrI)**	**DOR (95% CrI)**	**Mean % interpretable tests (range)**
Ophthalmoscopy	5	VCDR ≥ 0.7	60 (34-82)	94 (76-99)	26 (6-110)	98 (86-100)
Optic disc photography	6	VCDR ≥ 0.6	73 (61-83)	89 (50-99)	22 (3-148)	85(73-100)
RNFL photography	4	Diffuse and/ or localized defect	75 (46-92)	88 (53-98)	23 (4-124)	80
HRT II	3	≥ 1 Borderline or outside normal limits	86 (55-97)	89 (66-98)	51 (11-246)	94 (91-97)
FDTC-20-1	3	1 Abnormal point	92 (65-99)	94 (73-99)	181 (25-2139)	97 (87-99)
FDT C-20-5	5	1 Abnormal point	78 (19-99)	75 (57-87)	10 (0.7-249)	92 (86-98)
OKP	4	1 Abnormal point	86 (29-100)	90 (79-96)	58 (4-1585)	97 (94-98)
SAP suprathreshold	9	≥ 3 Points missing	71 (51-86)	85 (73-93)	14 (6-34)	81 (60-100)
SAP threshold	5	AGIS score ≥ 3	88 (65-97)	80 (55-93)	30 (6-159)	99 (91-100)
GAT	9	IOP > 21 mmHg	46 (22-71)	95 (89-97)	15 (4-49)	(90-100)

genetic markers could be used across different populations/ethnicities. The risk allele *Chromosome 7q31 risk allele (rs4236601A)* is commoner in both the POAG (28.7%) and non-glaucomatous controls (22.8%) and associated with a -modest increase in risk of POAG (Odds ratio: 1.36).[84] Both the low prevalence of disease causing mutations and the modest risk associated with more prevalent mutations limit the roles of genetic testing in screening for POAG.

Tests that measure contrast sensitivity, motion sensitivity, scotopic function, peripheral acuity, and other functions have been evaluated for glaucoma screening, but the results have been disappointing.[85]

6.9. Is glaucoma screening cost-effective?

Combining the tests mentioned in previous section and defining a positive screen as either test meeting the criterion of positivity can increase sensitivity. However, such an approach would lead to a concomitant loss of specificity because a non-diseased person would have two opportunities to produce a false-positive result. Such an approach may be desirable in a-clinic setting, but it is not justifiable from a cost-effective perspective for most population screening.

Vaahtoranta-Lehtonen *et al.*[60] modeled the cost effectiveness and cost utility of a screening program for glaucoma, in those aged 50-79, finding that one year of avoided visual disability was 32,000 euro, while the cost of one QALY gained by screening was estimated at 9,000 euro. Of interest, the cost of screening a population of 1 million was estimated at 30 million euro, producing 3,360 incremental QALY and 930 avoided years of disability for a total of 701 persons.

Burr *et al.*[16] in a systematic review concluded that general screening of the population at any age is not cost-effective, while selectively screening of groups with higher prevalence (such as family history, black ethnicity) might be worthwhile. Including less specific risk factors such as myopia and diabetes reduced the prevalence of POAG to the point that screening was not deemed cost-effective.

6.10. Does early detection of undiagnosed glaucoma matter?

The EMGT study, demonstrated that in a mixture of known cases and cases identified through screening, randomization into treatment vs. no treatment, led to a significant difference in the worsening of visual fields with those receiving treatment having better outcomes.[86] Similarly, in the United Kingdom Glaucoma

Treatment Study, those untreated developed worse visual fields than those treated. These large prospective RCTs provide convincing evidence that the combination of identifying and treating glaucoma cases, at least in a strict clinical trial setting, did make a difference in glaucoma progression, although it did not address the issue of preventing blindness, nor differences in quality of life. Likewise, the Collaborative Normal Tension Glaucoma Study (CNTGS) demonstrated that treatment slowed progression in this subset of patients.[87,88]

6.11. Tele-ophthalmology and glaucoma

Tele-ophthalmology mostly adopts the store-and-forward method, followed by interactive services and remote monitoring methods. The majority of the current tele-ophthalmology services concentrate on patient screening and appropriate referral to experts. Glaucoma management increasingly involves use of devices that are perceived to be 'telemedicine-friendly'. Automated perimetry, tonometry, corneal pachymetry, imaging of the optic disc, nerve fiber layer and anterior segment, may all generate digital outputs that can be transferred electronically and viewed remotely.[89]

A systematic review by Thomas *et al.* reported that tele-glaucoma is less sensitive (pooled sensitivity 83.2% [95% CI: 77%-88.1%] and more specific (pooled specificity 79% [95% CI: 66.8%-87.6%] than face-to-face clinical examination in detecting glaucoma.[90]

Wright et al described tele-glaucoma services in the UK supervised by a glaucoma specialist.[91] This is the largest tele-glaucoma study reported so far (24,257 patients). The mobile tele-team consisted of optometrists, technicians, diagnostic equipment, and support tools. There was good agreement (87%) between the optometrist and specialist, with a moderate κ value of 0.69. Of all those who were screened, only 0.054% were found to be at high risk by the specialist but were missed by optometrist.

6.12. Does screening reduce glaucoma related blindness and disability?

No data exist on this topic, and at present there are no active prospective studies registered to test this. A study of this nature might require more than a decade before any conclusive results could be found. In fact, Burr *et al.* studied this topic and concluded that a glaucoma screening trial in the UK is unlikely to be the best use of research resources.[92]

6.13. Conclusion

Issues such as the lack of a gold standard for glaucoma diagnosis, the difference in prevalence of disease in various populations, the challenge of performing screening in the general population, the cost of screening equipment and trained personnel, and the difficulties of providing access to the health care system to the screened patients, make screening for POAG a difficult undertaking in the present environment. Current consensus supports active case detection during eye evaluations and case finding among first degree relatives of known individuals with POAG. Improvements in screening technology or combined eye screening could lead to recommendations for broader screening of the population in the future.

References

1. Bourne RR, Stevens GA, White RA, et al.; the Vision Loss Expert Group. Causes of vision loss worldwide, 1990-2010: a systematic analysis. Lancet Glob Health 2013;1(6):e339-349.
2. Quigley HA, Broman A. The number of persons with glaucoma worldwide in 2010 and 2020. Br J Ophthalmol 2006;90:151-156.
3. Kim CS, Seong GJ, Lee NH, Song KC; the Namil Study Group, Korean Glaucoma Society. Prevalence of primary open-angle glaucoma in central South Korea the Namil study.Ophthalmology 2011;118(6):1024-1030.
4. Iwase A, Tomidokoro A, Araie M; the Tajimi Study Group of the Japan Glaucoma Society. Clinical Features of Undiagnosed Open Angle Glaucoma in Japan. Invest Ophthalmol Vis Sci 2006;47(13):3441.
5. Congdon N, O'Colmain B, Klaver CC, et al.; the Eye Diseases Prevalence Research Group. Causes and prevalence of visual impairment among adults in the United States. Arch Ophthalmol 2004;122(4):477-485.
6. Prum BE Jr, Rosenberg LF, Gedde SJ, et al. Primary Open-Angle Glaucoma Preferred Practice Pattern(®) Guidelines. Ophthalmology 2016;123(1):P41-P111.
7. Prum BE Jr, Herndon LW Jr, Moroi SE, et al. Primary Angle Closure Preferred Practice Pattern(®) Guidelines. Ophthalmology 2016;123(1):P1-P40.
8. Wilson JMG, Jungner G. Principles and Practice of Screening for Disease. WHO Chronicle 1968;22(11):473.
9. Quigley HA. Current and future approaches to glaucoma screening. J Glaucoma 1998;7(3):210-220.
10. Quigley HA, Addicks EM, Green R. Optic nerve damage in human glaucoma. Arch Ophthalmol 1982;100:135-146.
11. Harwerth RS, Carter-Dawson L, Shen F, Smith EL 3rd, Crawford ML. Ganglion cell losses underlying visual field defects from experimental glaucoma. Invest Ophthalmol Vis Sci 1999;40:2242-2250.
12. Schuman JS. Detection and Diagnosis of Glaucoma: Ocular Imaging. Invest Ophthalmol Vis Sci 2012;53(5):2488-2490.

13. Sommer A, Tielsch JM, Katz J, et al. Relationship between intraocular pressure and primary open angle glaucoma among white and black Americans. The Baltimore Eye Survey. Arch Ophthalmol 1991;109:1090-1095.
14. Quigley HA, West SK, Rodriguez J, et al. The prevalence of glaucoma in a population-based study of Hispanic subjects: Proyecto VER. Arch Ophthalmol 2001;119:1819-1826.
15. Farkas RH, Grosskreutz CL. Apoptosis, neuroprotection and retinal ganglion cell death: An overview. Int Ophthalmol Clin 2001;41:111-130.
16. Burr JM, Mowatt G, Hernández R, et al. The clinical effectiveness and cost-effectiveness of screening for open angle glaucoma: a systematic review and economic evaluation. Health Technol Assess 2007;11(41):iii-iv, ix-x,1-190.
17. Weinreb RN, Brandt JD, Garway-Heath D, Medeiros FA (Eds). Intraocular Pressure. World Glaucoma Association Consensus Series, no. 4. The Hague, The Netherlands: Kugler Publications 2007. http://www.worldglaucoma.org
18. Wang NL, Friedman DS, Zhou Q, Population-Based Assessment of 24-Hour Intraocular Pressure among Subjects with Primary Open-Angle Glaucoma: The Handan Eye Study. Invest Ophthalmol Vis Sci 2011;52(11):7817-7821.
19. Kass MA, Heuer DK, Higginbotham EJ, et al.; the Ocular Hypertension Treatment Study Group. The Ocular Hypertension Treatment Study. A randomized trial determines that topical ocular hypotensive medication delays or prevents the onset of primary open-angle glaucoma. Arch Ophthalmol 2002;120:701-713.
20. Hattenhauer MG, Johnson DH, Ing HH, et al. The probability of blindness from open-angle glaucoma. Ophthalmology 1998;105:2099-2104.
21. The Advanced Glaucoma Intervention Study (AGIS): 12. Baseline risk factors for sustained loss of visual field and visual acuity in patients with advanced glaucoma. Am J Ophthalmol 2002;134(4):499-512.
22. Fong DS, Epstein DL, Allingham RR. Glaucoma and myopia: are they related? Int Ophthalmol Clin 1990;30(3):215-218.
23. Knapp A. Glaucoma in Myopic Eyes. Trans Am Ophthalmol Soc 1925;23:61-70.
24. Podos SM, Becker B, Morton WR. High myopia and primary open-angle glaucoma. Am J Ophthalmol 1966;62(6):1038-1043.
25. Abdalla MI, Hamdi M. Applanation ocular tension in myopia and emmetropia. Br J Ophthalmol 1970;54(2):122-125.
26. Perkins ES, Phelps CD. Open angle glaucoma, ocular hypertension, low-tension glaucoma, and refraction. Arch Ophthalmol 1982;100(9):1464-1467.
27. Daubs JG, Crick RP Effect of refractive error on the risk of ocular hypertension and open angle glaucoma. Trans Ophthalmol Soc U K, 1981;101(1):121-126.
28. Gordon MO, Beiser JA, Brandt JD, et al. The Ocular Hypertension Treatment Study: baseline factors that predict the onset of primary open angle glaucoma. Arch Ophthalmol 2002;120(6):714-720; discussion 829-830.
29. Qiu M, Wang SY, Singh K, Lin SC. Association between Myopia and Glaucoma in the United States Population. Invest Ophthalmol Vis Sci 2013;54(1):830-835.
30. Xu L, Wang Y, Wang S, Wang Y, Jonas JB. High myopia and glaucoma susceptibility the Beijing Eye Study. Ophthalmology 2007;114(2):216-220.
31. Perera SA, Wong TY, Tay W-T, et al. Refractive Error, Axial Dimensions and Primary Open Angle Glaucoma: The Singapore Malay Eye Study. Arch Ophthalmol 2010;128(7):900-905.

32. Kim KE, Kim MJ, Park KH, et al.; the Epidemiologic Survey Committee of the Korean Ophthalmological Society. Prevalence, Awareness, and Risk Factors of Primary Open-Angle Glaucoma: Korea National Health and Nutrition Examination Survey 2008-2011. Ophthalmology 2015 Dec 30. [Epub ahead of print]
33. Chang RT, Singh K. Myopia and glaucoma: diagnostic and therapeutic challenges. Curr Opin Ophthalmol 2013;24:96-101.
34. Mwanza JC, Sayyad FE, Aref AA, et al. Rates of abnormal retinal nerve fiber layer and ganglion cell layer OCT scans in healthy myopic eyes: cirrus versus RTVue. Ophthalmic Surg Lasers Imaging 2012;43(6 Suppl):S67-74.
35. Leske MC, Wu SY, Hennis A, Honkanen R, Nemesure B; the BESs Study Group. Risk factors for incident open-angle glaucoma: the Barbados Eye Studies. Ophthalmology 2008;115(1):85-93.
36. de Voogd S, Ikram MK, Wolfs RC, Jansonius NM, Hofman A, de Jong PT. Incidence of open-angle glaucoma in a general elderly population: the Rotterdam Study. Ophthalmology 2005;112(9):1487-1493.
37. Wensor MD, McCarty CA, Stanislavsky YL, Livingston PM, Taylor HR. The prevalence of glaucoma in the Melbourne Visual Impairment Project. Ophthalmology 1998;105(4):733-739.
38. Kosoko-Lasaki O, Gong G, Haynatzki G, Wilson MR. Race, ethnicity and prevalence of primary open-angle glaucoma. J Natl Med Assoc 2006;98(10):1626-1629.
39. Chan EW, Li X, Tham YC, et al. Glaucoma in Asia: regional prevalence variations and future projections. Br J Ophthalmol 2016;100(1):78-85.
40. Sommer A. Glaucoma risk factors observed in the Baltimore Eye Survey. Curr Opin Ophthalmol 1996;7(2):93-98.
41. Wolfs RC, Klaver CC, Ramrattan RS, et al. Genetic risk of primary open-angle glaucoma. Population-based familial aggregation study. Arch Ophthalmol 1998;116(12):1640-1645.
42. Sung VCT, Koppens JM, Vernon SA, et al. Longitudinal glaucoma screening for siblings of patients with primary open angle glaucoma: the Nottingham Family Glaucoma Screening Study. Br J Ophthalmol 2006;90(1):59-63.
43. Abu-Amero K, Kondkar AA, Chalam KV. An Updated Review on the Genetics of Primary Open Angle Glaucoma. Int J Mol Sci 2015;16(12):28886-28911.
44. Liu Y, Hauser MA, Akafo SK, et al. Investigation of Known Genetic Risk Factors for Primary Open Angle Glaucoma in Two Populations of African Ancestry. Invest Ophthalmol Vis Sci 2013;54(9): 6248-6254.
45. Chung HJ, Hwang HB, Lee NY. The Association between Primary Open-Angle Glaucoma and Blood Pressure: Two Aspects of Hypertension and Hypotension. Biomed Res Int 2015;2015:827516.
46. Zhou M, Wang W, Huang W, Zhang X. Diabetes Mellitus as a Risk Factor for Open-Angle Glaucoma: A Systematic Review and Meta-Analysis. PLoS One 2014;9(8):e102972.
47. Phelps CD, Corbett JJ. Migraine and low-tension glaucoma. A case-control study. Invest Ophthalmol Vis Sci 1985;26(8):1105-1108.
48. Jost B. Jonas, Ningli Wang. Cerebrospinal Fluid Pressure and Glaucoma. J Ophthalmic Vis Res 2013;8(3):257-263.
49. Gillow JT, Shah P, O'Neill EC. Primary open angle glaucoma and hypothyroidism: Chance or true association? Eye 1997;11:113-114.
50. Khandgave TP, Puthran N, Ingole AB, Nicholson AD. The Assessment of Sleep Apnoea as a Risk Factor in Glaucoma. J Clin Diagn Res 2013;7(7):1391-1393.

51. Gramlich OW, Beck S, von Thun und Hohenstein-Blaul N, et al. Enhanced Insight into the Autoimmune Component of Glaucoma: IgG Autoantibody Accumulation and Pro-Inflammatory Conditions in Human Glaucomatous Retina. PLoS One 2013;8(2):e57557.
52. Križaj D, Ryskamp DA, Tian N, et al. From Mechanosensitivity to Inflammatory Responses: New Players in the Pathology of Glaucoma. Curr Eye Res 2014;39(2):105-119.
53. Medeiros FA, Weinreb RN, Sample PA, et al. Validation of a Predictive Model to Estimate the Risk of Conversion From Ocular Hypertension to Glaucoma. Arch Ophthalmol 2005;123(10):1351-1360.
54. Francis BA, Varma R, Vigen C, et al.; the Los Angeles Latino Eye Study Group. Population and High-Risk Group Screening for Glaucoma: The Los Angeles Latino Eye Study. Invest Ophthalmol Vis Sci 2011;52(9):6257-6264.
55. Rudnicka AR, Mt-Isa S, Owen CG, Cook DG, Ashby D. Variations in primary open-angle glaucoma prevalence by age, gender, and race: a Bayesian meta-analysis. Invest Ophthalmol Vis Sci 2006;47(10):4254-4261.
56. Hatt S, Wormald R, Burr J. Screening for prevention of optic nerve damage due to chronic open angle glaucoma. Cochrane Database Syst Rev 2006;(4):CD006129.
57. Gottlieb LK, Schwartz B, Pauker SG.Glaucoma screening. A cost-effectiveness analysis. Survey of Ophthalmology 1983;3:206-226.
58. Hernández RA, Burr JM, Vale LD; OAG Screening Project Group. Economic evaluation of screening for open-angle glaucoma. Int J Technol Assess Health Care 2008;24(2):203-211.
59. Boivin JF, McGregor M, Archer C. Cost effectiveness of screening for primary open angle glaucoma. J Med Screen 1996;3(3):154-163.
60. Vaahtoranta-Lehtonen H, Tuulonen A, Aronen P. Cost effectiveness and cost utility of an organized screening programme for glaucoma. Acta Ophthalmol Scand 2007;85(5):508-518.
61. Hoskins HD Jr. Glaucoma care cost-effectiveness. Ophthalmology 2009;116(5):1016.
62. Weinreb RN, Healey PR, Topouzis F. (Eds.). Glaucoma Screening. World Glaucoma Association Consensus Series, no. 5. The Hague, The Netherlands: Kugler Publications 2008.
63. Salim S, Netland PA, Fung KH, et al. Assessment of the Student Sight Savers Program methods for glaucoma screening. Ophthalmic Epidemiol 2009;16(4):238-242.
64. Dandona L, Dandona R, Srinivas M, et al. Open angle glaucoma in an urban population in southern India: the Andhra Pradesh Eye Disease Study. Ophthalmology 2000;107:1702-1709.
65. Raychaudhuri A, Lahiri SK, Bandyopadhyay M, et al. A population based survey of the prevalence and types of glaucoma in rural West Bengal: The West Bengal Glaucoma Study. Br J Ophthalmol 2005;89:1559-1564.
66. Kapetanakis VV, Chan MPY, Foster PJ, et al. Global variations and time trends in the prevalence of primary open angle glaucoma (POAG): a systematic review and meta-analysis. Brit J Ophthalmol 2016;100(1):86-93.
67. Harper R, Radi N, Reeves BC, et al. Agreement between ophthalmologists and optometrists in optic disc assessment: training implications for glaucoma co-management. Graefes Arch Clin Exp Ophthalmol 2001;239(5):342-350.
68. Abrams LS, Scott IU, Spaeth GL, Quigley HA, Varma R. Agreement among optometrists, ophthalmologists, and residents in evaluating the optic disc for glaucoma. Ophthalmology 1994;101(10):1662-1667.
69. Bennett R, Spry PG, Fenerty CH, Harper RA. Technical Note: grading the vertical cup:disc ratio and the effect of scaling. Ophthalmic Physiol Opt 2007;27(6):619-625.

70. Chan HH, Ong DN, Kong YX, et al. Glaucomatous optic neuropathy evaluation (GONE) project: the effect of monoscopic versus stereoscopic viewing conditions on optic nerve evaluation. Am J Ophthalmol 2014;157(5):936-944.
71. Waisbourd M, Bond EA, Sullivan T, et al. Evaluation of Nonmydriatic Hand-held Optic Disc Photography Grading in the Philadelphia Glaucoma Detection and Treatment Project. J Glaucoma 2016;25(5):e520-525.
72. Lai JS, Gangwani RA. Medication-induced acute angle closure attack. Hong Kong Med J 2012;18(2):139-145.
73. Ervin AM, Boland MV, Myrowitz EH, et al. Screening for Glaucoma: Comparative Effectiveness [Internet]. Rockville (MD): Agency for Healthcare Research and Quality (US); 2012 Apr. (Comparative Effectiveness Reviews, No. 59.) Results. Available from: http://www.ncbi.nlm.nih.gov/books/NBK95377/
74. Healey PR, Lee AJ, Aung T, et al. Diagnostic accuracy of the Heidelberg Retina Tomograph for Glaucoma: a population-based assessment. Ophthalmology 2010;117:1667-1674.
75. Saito H, Tsutsumi T, Araie M, et al. Sensitivity and specificity of the Heidelberg Retina Tomograph II version 3.0 in a population-based study: The Tajimi Study. Ophthalmology 2009;116:1854-1861.
76. Balendra SI, Normando EM, Bloom PA, Cordeiro MF. Advances in retinal ganglion cell imaging. Eye (Lond) 2015;29(10):1260-1269.
77. Li G, Fansi AK, Boivin JF, et al. Screening for glaucoma in high-risk populations using optical coherence tomography. Ophthalmology 2010;117:453-461.
78. Bengtsson B, Andersson S, Heijl A. Performance of time-domain and spectral-domain Optical Coherence Tomography for glaucoma screening. Acta Ophthalmol 2010;90:310-315.
79. North RV, Jones AL, Hunter E, Morgan JE, Wild JM. Evaluation of the high specificity Screening Program (C-20-1) of the Frequency Doubling Technology (FDT) perimeter in clinical practice. Eye (Lond) 2006;20(6):681-687.
80. Mowatt G, Burr JM, Cook JA, et al. Screening Tests for Detecting Open-Angle Glaucoma: Systematic Review and Meta-analysis. Invest Ophthalmol Vis Sci 2008;49(12):5373-5385.
81. Francis BA, Varma R, Vigen C, et al. Population and High-Risk Group Screening for Glaucoma: The Los Angeles Latino Eye Study. Invest Ophthalmol Vis Sci 2011;52(9):6257-6264.
82. Michelessi M, Lucenteforte E, Oddone F, et al. Optic nerve head and fibre layer imaging for diagnosing glaucoma. Cochrane Database of Systematic Reviews 2015;11. Art. No.: CD008803.
83. Fingert JH. Primary open-angle glaucoma genes. Eye 2011;25(5):587-595.
84. Kuehn MH, Wang K, Roos B, et al. Chromosome 7q31 POAG locus: ocular expression of caveolins and lack of association with POAG in a US cohort. Molecular Vision 2011;17:430-435.
85. Graham SL, Drance SM, Chauhan BC, et al. Comparison of psychophysical and electrophysiological testing in early glaucoma. Invest Ophthalmol Vis Sci 1996;37(13):2651-2662.
86. Garway-Heath DF, Crabb DP, Bunce C, et al. Latanoprost for open-angle glaucoma (UKGTS): a randomised, multicentre, placebo-controlled trial. Lancet 2015;385(9975):1295-1304. Erratum in: Lancet 2015;386(9989):136.
87. The effectiveness of intraocular pressure reduction in the treatment of normal-tension glaucoma. Collaborative Normal-Tension Glaucoma Study Group. Am J Ophthalmol 1998;126(4):498-505.
88. Krupin T, Liebmann JM, Greenfield DS, et al.; the Low-Pressure Glaucoma Study Group. TheLow-pressure Glaucoma Treatment Study (LoGTS) study design and baseline characteristics of enrolled patients. Ophthalmology 2005;112(3):376-385.

89. Kiage D, Kherani IN, Gichuhi S, Damji KF, Nyenze M. The Muranga Teleophthalmology Study: Comparison of Virtual (Teleglaucoma) with in-Person Clinical Assessment to Diagnose Glaucoma. Middle East Afr J Ophthalmol 2013;20(2):150-157.
90. Thomas SM, Jeyaraman MM, Hodge WG, et al. The Effectiveness of Teleglaucoma versus In-Patient Examination for Glaucoma Screening: A Systematic Review and Meta-Analysis. PLoS One 2014;9(12):e113779.
91. Wright HR, Diamond JP. Service innovation in glaucoma management: using a web-based electronic patient record to facilitate virtual specialist supervision of a shared care glaucoma programme. Br J Ophthalmol 2015;99:313-317.
92. Burr J, Hernández R, Ramsay C, et al. Is it worthwhile to conduct a randomized controlled trial of glaucoma screening in the United Kingdom? J Health Serv Res Pol 2014;19(1):42-51.

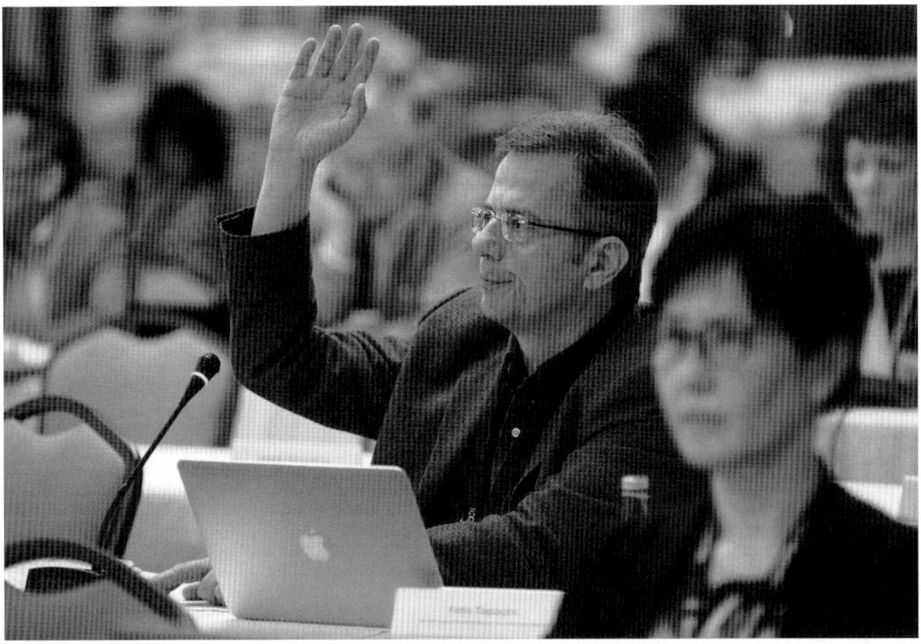

Fotis Topouzis

SUMMARY CONSENSUS POINTS

Section 1 - Structure

1. Clinical evaluation and documentation of the optic nerve head is essential for the diagnosis and the monitoring of glaucoma.
2. Clinical diagnosis of glaucoma is predicated on the detection of a thinned retinal nerve fiber layer (RNFL) and narrowed neuroretinal rim.

   Comments: These features often are accompanied by deformation of the optic nerve head (ONH) (cupping).

   These features often appear first in the supero- or inferotemporal quadrants.

   Although these features are characteristic of POAG, it is important to exclude non-glaucomatous optic neuropathies.
3. Detecting progressive glaucomatous RNFL thinning and neuroretinal rim narrowing are the best currently available gold standards for glaucoma diagnosis.

   Comment: Disease-related damage should be differentiated from age-related change.
4. The diagnosis of glaucoma does not always require the detection of visual field defects with perimetry.

   Comments: Perimetric defects that correspond to structural findings increase the likelihood of glaucoma.

   Perimetry is indispensable for documentation and monitoring of functional decline in glaucoma.
5. Assessment of the color and the configuration (size and shape) of the neuroretinal rim is important to differentiate glaucomatous from non-glaucomatous optic neuropathies.

   Comment: A pale rim suggests non-glaucomatous optic neuropathy.
6. Photography is effective to document glaucomatous optic disc appearance and nerve fiber layer damage.

   Comments: Photography is particularly useful for detecting and documenting optic disc hemorrhage and rim color.

   Stereophotography is particularly useful for documenting optic disc topography.
7. Imaging technologies including optical coherence tomography (OCT), confocal scanning laser ophthalmoscopy (CSLO) and scanning laser polarimetry (SLP) provide an objective and quantitative approach to detect and monitor glaucoma.

8. OCT may be the best currently available digital imaging instrument for detecting and tracking optic nerve structural damage in glaucoma.
9. RNFL thickness is the most clinically helpful parameter of the ones currently available with OCT.
   Comments: Macular RGC loss in glaucoma also can be detected by OCT.
   RNFL thickness and macular RGC loss are complementary.
   Pitfalls of OCT such as artifacts and false segmentation should be considered when using OCT.
   GCIPL thickness (macula): The macula has the highest density of RGCs.
10. It is difficult in myopic eyes to differentiate those with and without glaucoma.
    Comments: In myopic eyes, documented progressive optic neuropathy can be used to make the differential diagnosis of glaucoma.
    Reference databases do not currently include highly myopic eyes and, therefore, are not appropriate for diagnosing RNFL damage in them.

Section 2- Vision function

1. Functional testing is essential for the evaluation, staging and monitoring of glaucoma
   Comment: Standard automated perimetry (SAP) is the reference standard for all functional testing.
2. Clinical decisions should be made based on reliable visual field tests.
   Comments: Visual field defects should be reproducible and/or should be consistent with the location of the optic nerve defects.
   The most important reliability criterion is the false positive rate.
3. In the presence of glaucomatous optic neuropathy, a Glaucoma Hemifield Test (GHT) 'outside normal limits' in a reliable visual field indicates that glaucomatous visual field loss is present.
   Comment: For instruments not calculating a GHT, an abnormal ($P < 5\%$) pattern standard deviation (PSD) or square-root-loss variance (sLV) likely have similar diagnostic value.
4. When glaucomatous optic neuropathy (GON) is suspected, a GHT criterion of 'outside normal limits' or 'borderline' in a reliable visual field increases the probability that an eye has glaucoma.
   Comment: The level of probability for glaucoma depends on the presence and magnitude of other risk factors for glaucoma (such as raised intraocular pressure) and the quality of evidence that there is no GON.

5. Before a visual field defect can be confirmed as glaucomatous, retinal and non-glaucomatous optic disc conditions should be excluded by a careful examination of the retina and optic disc.
   Comment: If the pattern of visual field loss suggests a neurological origin, or if there is incongruity between the pattern of visual field loss and optic disc and retinal nerve fiber layer appearance, then further investigation is warranted (*e.g.*, color vision testing, neuroimaging).
6. Standard white-on-white automated perimetry (SAP), with a fixed testing matrix covering at least the central 24 degrees, is preferred for the diagnosis of glaucomatous visual field loss.
   Comments: Goldmann size III stimuli are conventionally used in most automated perimeters in clinical practice for glaucoma diagnosis.
   For more severe cases size V, increases the dynamic range and reduces variability of test results.
   Using the 10-2 strategy, in addition to the conventional 24-2 Humphrey grid, can improve the detection of central functional loss
7. Threshold algorithms are preferred over supra-threshold algorithms for glaucoma diagnosis.
   Comment: Supra-threshold algorithms can be helpful in cases of unreliable results from threshold testing algorithms.
8. Neither short-wavelength automated perimetry (SWAP) nor frequency doubling technology (FDT) perimetry have superior diagnostic precision to SAP.
   Comments: Patients should be followed consistently with same visual function test and ideally one with statistical support for recognizing change.
   The more diagnostic tests that are performed, the more likely it is that one will be 'outside normal limits', therefore increasing the number of false positive results.
9. Patients who are at risk for glaucoma and have normal standard automated perimetry (SAP) should have their visual function monitored to detect deterioration and hence establish a glaucoma diagnosis.
   Comment: The earliest evidence for glaucoma may be functional or structural. Therefore, both should be measured to ensure that the onset of glaucoma damage is not overlooked.
10. Deterioration may be first detected by the glaucoma hemifield test (GHT) (or summary parameters) or by trend analysis of measurements over time. Which analysis is most sensitive varies between patients and so both should be done.

7. As yet there is no widely-accepted method of combining the results of structural and functional tests.
   Comment: Several proposed methods for combining structural and/or functional measurements offer advantages over traditional parameters and continue to be investigated.
8. Physicians should be aware of false-positive tests and over-diagnosing glaucoma, which are more likely when using a large number of diagnostic tests.
   Comment: Although using multiple parameters may increase overall diagnostic sensitivity, the chance will also increase of falsely labeling a change significant.

Section 4 - Risk factors (ocular)

1. Although POAG may develop at any IOP, there is strong evidence supporting higher mean intraocular pressure during follow-up as a risk factor for development and progression of glaucomatous damage.
   Comments: There is insufficient evidence and further studies are needed to elucidate which IOP parameter(s) (mean, peak and/or fluctuation, area under IOP curve, etc.) is most important in determining risk of glaucoma development or progression.
   There is insufficient evidence implicating IOP fluctuations as an independent risk factor for glaucoma development or progression.
2. Low ocular perfusion pressure (OPP) (the difference between systemic blood pressure and intraocular pressure) is associated with increased prevalence of open-angle glaucoma in cross-sectional studies.
   Comments: The value of OPP monitoring in daily clinical practice is not established.
   Due to the intrinsic relationship between OPP and IOP, it is difficult to establish an independent contribution of OPP as a risk factor for the development of glaucoma.
3. There is insufficient evidence supporting the role of provocative tests, such as the water-drinking test, as providing independent contribution to assess risk of glaucoma development and progression.
   Comment: Prospective longitudinal studies are necessary to clarify whether the water-drinking provocative test can provide additional information over office-based IOP measurements in establishing risk of glaucoma development or progression.

4. There is strong evidence supporting the role of central corneal thickness (CCT) as an important predictive factor for glaucoma development in ocular hypertensives and glaucoma suspects. Baseline CCT measurements should be obtained in patients suspected of having glaucoma.
   Comments: Algorithms to correct IOP based on CCT measurements are not recommended for routine use in clinical practice.
   There is insufficient evidence to conclude whether or not CCT is a true independent risk factor for glaucoma development or progression, or whether its effect is related to a tonometric artifact.
   There is no evidence that serial CCT measurements have value in clinical evaluation glaucoma.
5. There is strong evidence implicating lower corneal hysteresis as a risk factor for glaucoma development and progression.
   Comments: There is insufficient evidence about the mechanisms by which corneal hysteresis is associated with risk of glaucoma progression.
6. Existing evidence suggests that individuals with myopia have an increased risk of developing open angle glaucoma, with the risk being greater for people with high myopia.
   Comments: Diagnosis of glaucoma among myopic eyes can be challenging. Confirmed evidence of glaucomatous progression from a well-defined baseline is important for a correct diagnosis in many myopic individuals.
7. Disc hemorrhage is associated with increased risk of developing glaucoma and it is a marker for glaucomatous progression.
   Comment: Consideration of treatment escalation or closer follow-up should be given for patients presenting with optic disc hemorrhages.
8. Predictive models (risk calculators) may provide objective assessment of individual risk and their use should be considered in patients suspected of having glaucoma.
   Comment: Current validated risk calculators apply only to OHT patients. Moreover, they do not include all known risk factors.

Section 5 - Risk assessment

1. Primary open-angle glaucoma (POAG) occurs at all ages, and the incidence and prevalence accelerates with age.
2. Populations with the highest incidence and prevalence of POAG have African ancestry.

Comment: Due to the earlier age of disease onset, the average duration of POAG may be greatest in individuals of African ancestry.

3. Hispanics may have higher incidence and prevalence of POAG than individuals of European ancestry (non-Hispanic whites).
4. Older age is a risk factor for glaucoma onset and progression.
5. Although an increased prevalence of POAG in men has been reported, there is not enough evidence to support an association of POAG risk with male gender.
6. Lower socioeconomic status may be associated with later presentation of POAG.
7. First-degree relatives of POAG patients are at higher risk for glaucoma.
8. Although genetic association studies have revealed multiple associated loci for POAG, there is little value for routine genetic testing to diagnose or predict the development of glaucoma at the current time.
9. There is consistent, but weak, positive association between diastolic blood pressure and IOP and between systolic blood pressure and IOP in population-based studies.
10. Lower blood pressure (BP) and ocular perfusion pressure are associated with higher glaucoma prevalence and incidence across all racial groups.
    Comment: It is not known whether ocular perfusion pressure (OPP) is an independent risk factor for glaucoma due to the fact that IOP is intrinsically used in the calculation as performed with current methods.
11. The relationships between diastolic blood pressure, systolic blood pressure, systemic hypotension or systemic hypertension, and POAG are inconsistent.
12. The relationship between treatment of systemic hypertension and the development of POAG remains unclear.
    Comment: There are data suggesting that some patients being treated for systemic hypertension may be at greater risk for development of POAG.
13. The role of nocturnal systemic hypotension in the development of glaucoma is not known.
14. The evidence that obstructive sleep apnea is a risk factor for open-angle glaucoma (OAG) is weak and warrants further study.
15. Diabetes mellitus likely increases the risk for glaucoma onset.
16. There is insufficient evidence to determine if thyroid disease is associated with glaucoma.
17. Although there is some evidence that reduction of estrogen production in post-menopausal women increases glaucoma risk, there is insufficient evidence for hormonal replacement.

Section 6 - Screening

1. Glaucoma is the leading cause of irreversible blindness worldwide.
   Comment: In some countries, as many as 90% of glaucoma patients remain undiagnosed.
2. Screening everyone for glaucoma is an ideal proposition, but it is not logistically feasible. It would also result in an unacceptably high number of individuals with a false-positive diagnosis of glaucoma.
   Comment: To be effective, screening programs should select participants at substantial risk for glaucoma.
3. The cost-effectiveness of screening for POAG alone has not been demonstrated.
   Comment: Cost-effectiveness for glaucoma may be enhanced when done with other ocular conditions that cause visual impairment, including uncorrected refractive error, cataract, diabetic retinopathy, and age-related macular degeneration.
4. First-degree relatives of individuals with POAG and those with significant risk factors should be examined.

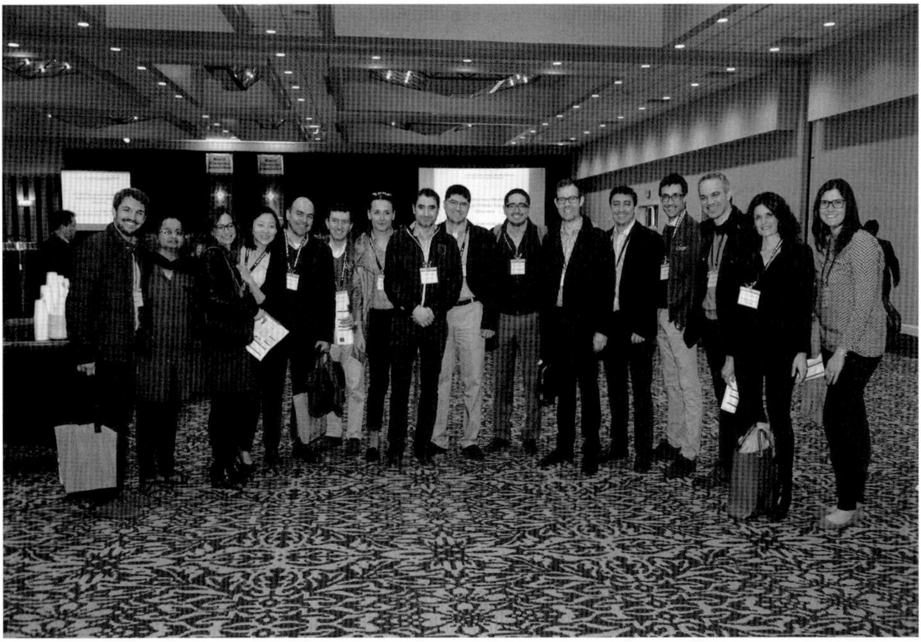

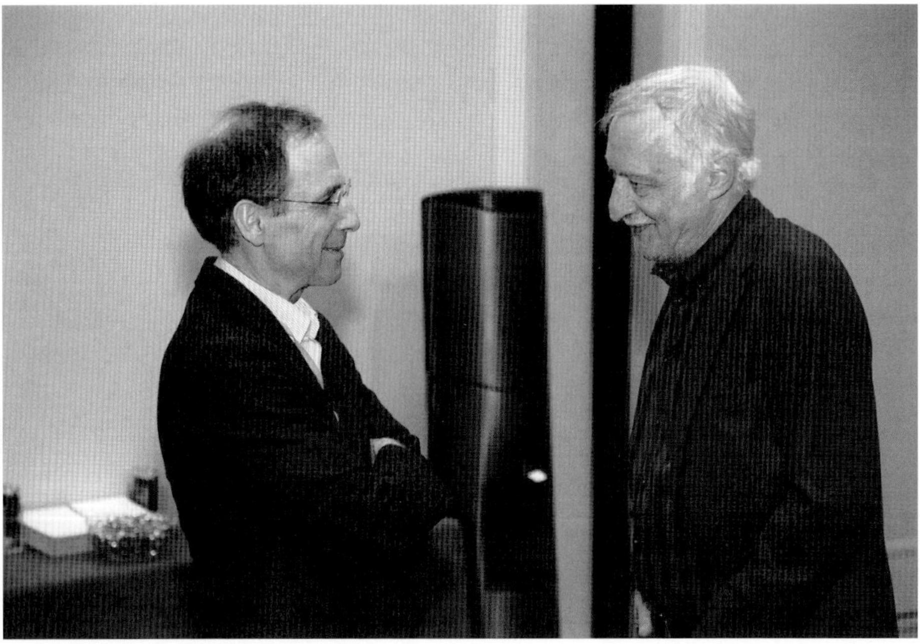

Norbert Pfeiffer and Gerhard Zinsser

CONSENSUS AND THE WORLD GLAUCOMA ASSOCIATION

As providing education is one the core goals of the WGA, IGR is one of the key pillars of the WGA Educational activities. Below we provide you with an overview of the WGA purpose, core values and goals.

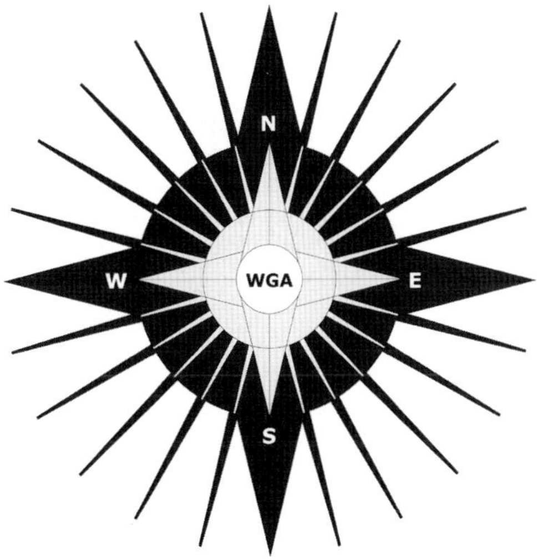

WGA core purpose

To eliminate glaucoma-related disability worldwide.

WGA core values

The leadership and member societies of WGA are committed to acting consistently with the following values:

- Responsibility (Accountability) – to each other, to member societies, to the larger global glaucoma community, to the patient and to the public.
- Consensus – open communication, inclusion of diverse viewpoints, and the aspiration to achieve practical consensus before acting.
- Collegiality and Mutual Respect.
- Best Care and Service – advancing the best care available to glaucoma patients worldwide.

WGA strategic goals

1. Education: The WGA will be an important source of education for ophthalmologists and other healthcare providers related to glaucoma.
2. WGC: The WGC will be the best glaucoma meeting in the world.
3. Public Awareness and Recognition of Glaucoma: Public awareness and recognition of glaucoma will increase.
4. Impact in Developing Countries: The resources of the global glaucoma community—including individuals, member societies, industry, governments, NGOs and patients—will be integrated and leveraged to enhance glaucoma care, particularly in developing countries.
5. Technology: The WGA will use information/communication technologies as a key tool in achieving its goals.
6. Organization: The WGA will be financially sound and organized to lead the glaucoma community.

More information about WGA is available via www.worldglaucoma.org

WGA contact details:

WGA Executive Office
Schipluidenlaan 4
1062 HE Amsterdam
The Netherlands
T: +31 20 679 3411
E: info@worldglaucoma.org

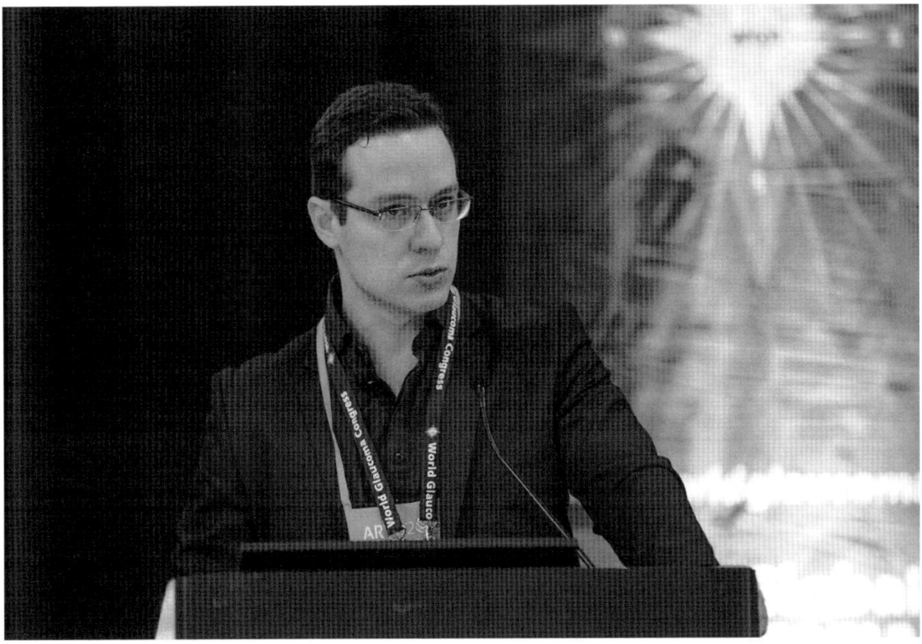

Gustavo DeMoraes

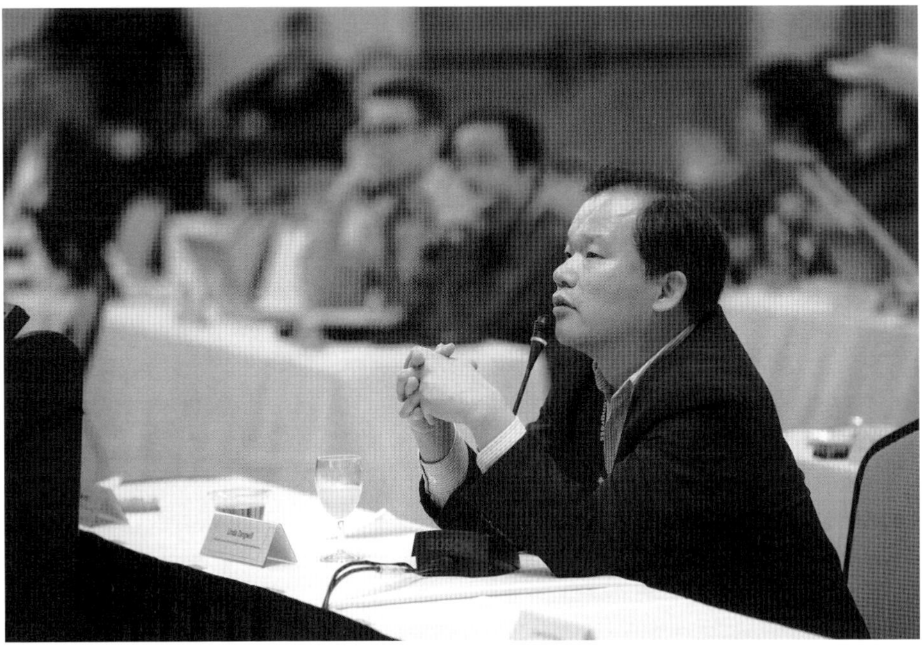

Tae Woo Kim

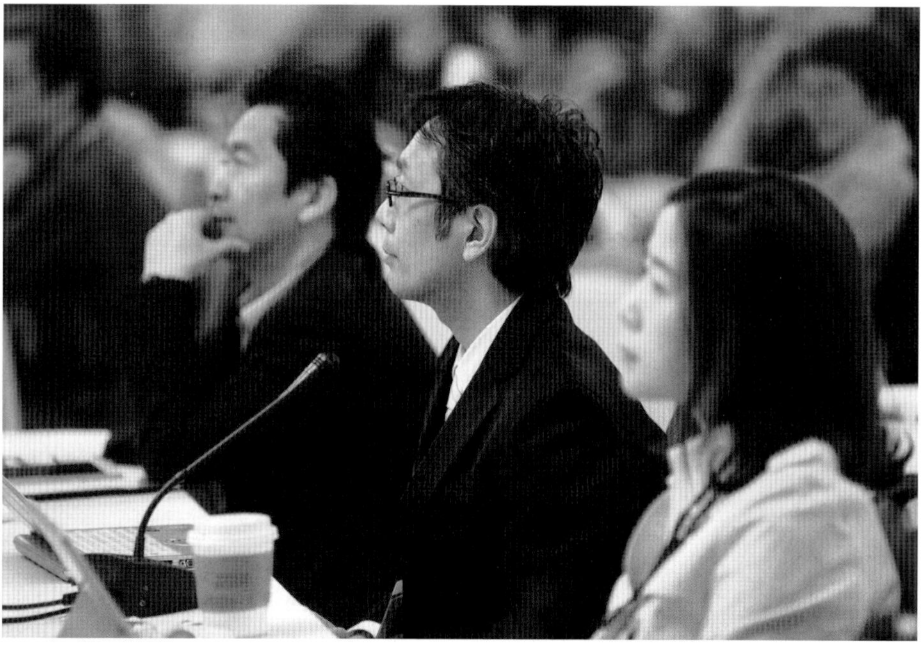

Toru Nakasawa and Miki Atsuya

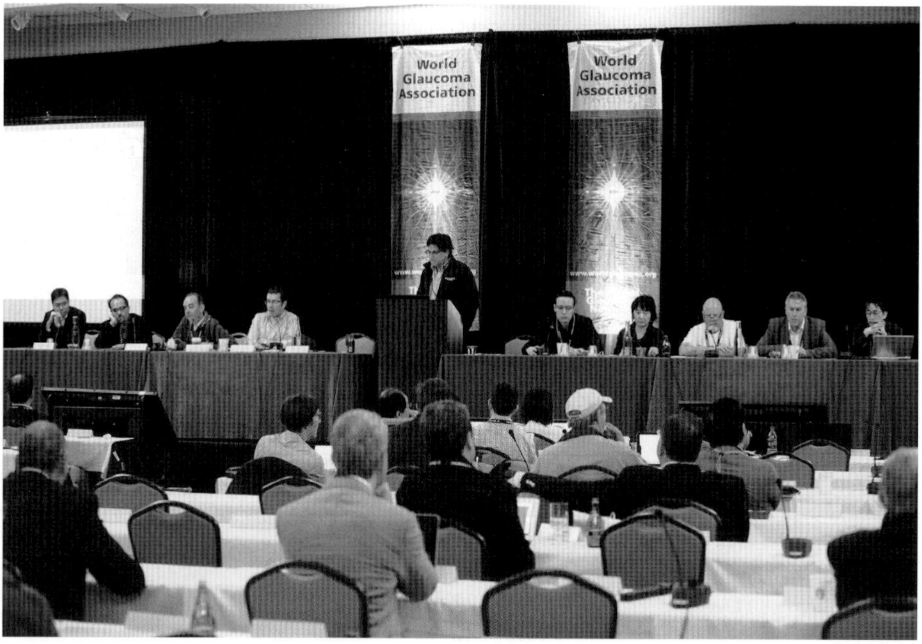

Chris Leung, Felipe Medeiros, Jeff Liebmann, David Garway-Heath and Robert N. Weinreb

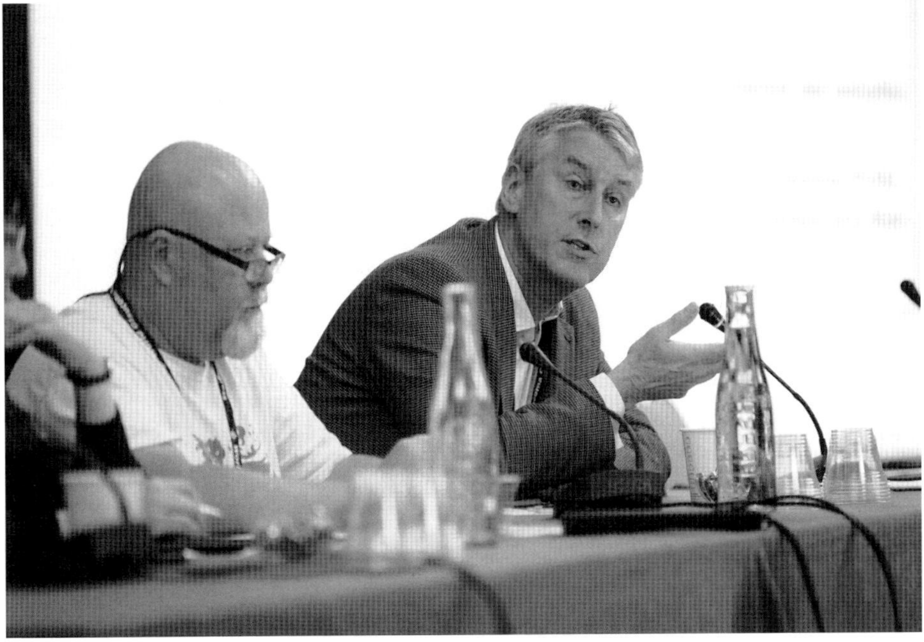

Chris Bowd and Andrew McNaught

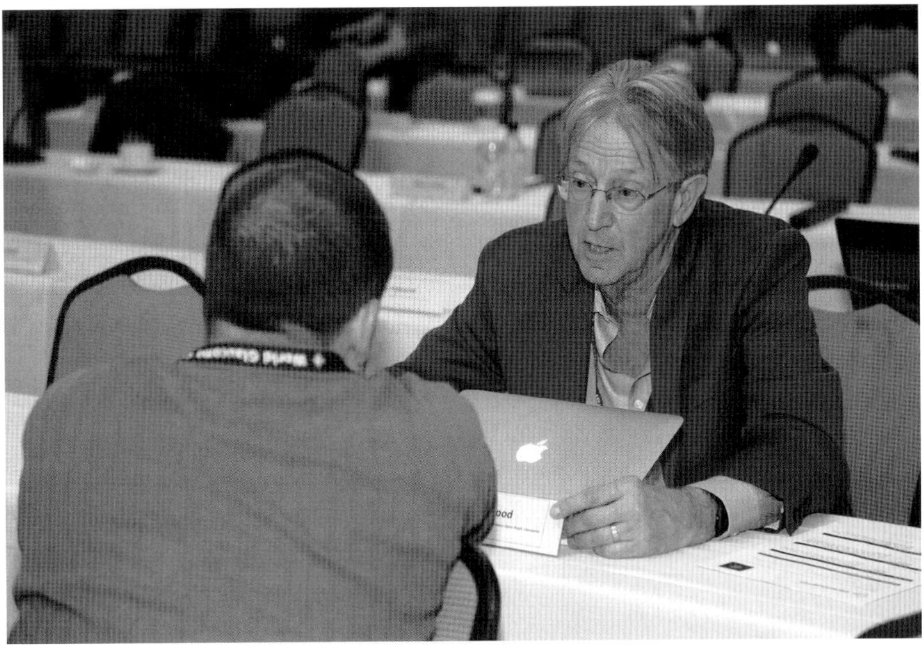

Don Hood

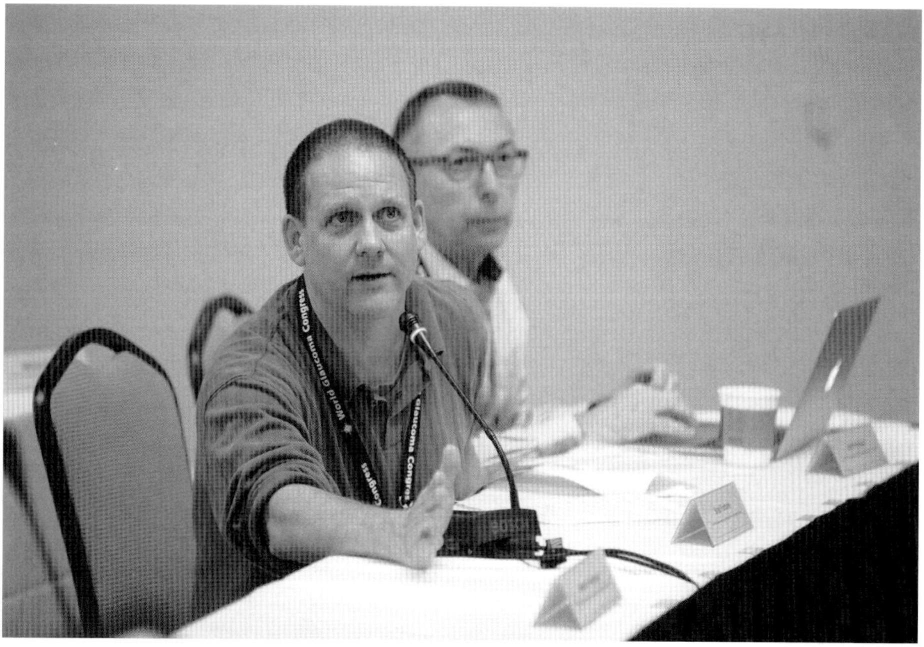

Brad Fortune and John Flanagan

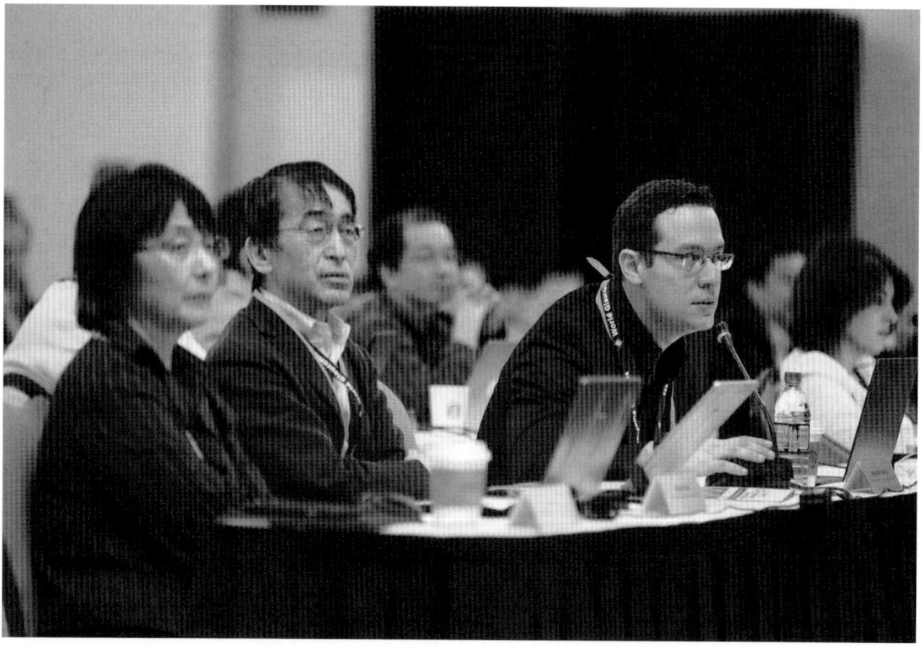

Aiko Iwase, Makoto Araie and Gustavo De Moraes

INDEX OF AUTHORS

NOTES

NOTES

NOTES

NOTES